SECOND WIND

Thriving with Cancer

SECOND WIND

Thriving with Cancer

DANN WONSER, MA, LPC

WHAT PEOPLE ARE SAYING ABOUT SECOND WIND

This is one of the most thoughtful and useful books I've read, and certainly a must-read for anyone in the health professions. This narrative will help health professionals learn to provide more supportive, compassionate, and collaborative care.

Beyond that, it is an amazing book for any of us trying to live consciously on this planet. Dann gives step by step, humorous, compassionate, and practical instructions for what worked for him to move towards becoming his best self.

I loved reading this!!! I laughed out loud!

~ Dawn Doutrich, PhD, RN, CNS Emeritus
Washington State University College of Nursing

There is a rare intimacy as Dann leads readers through his cancer journey. The book is hard to put down. As a survivor I found myself saying, "I felt that, too!"

The book provided a way for me to reflect on how I handled fear, anger, and a host of other issues. By the end of the book I was asking, how did cancer lead me back to myself?

~ Charlotte de Renne, Cancer Survivor

Dann is an extraordinary writer. He has clarity of thought and a level of introspection that rings true.

~Sandip Patel, MD, Oncologist, UCSD Moores Cancer Center

This book is engaging, thought provoking and emotionally charged. Learning to meet and accept life with joy on life's terms is no small task. From the plethora of emotions to managing relationships, and from fighting the stigma to becoming your own health care advocate, the writer shows us his roadmap.

I commend this writer for sharing his journey with truth.

~ Bill Hogan, Cancer Caregiver

~

100 percent of the net profits from this book will be donated to the two lung cancer advocacy/support organizations below. I have the greatest of respect, and owe an enormous debt of gratitude, to both. They have enriched the lives of everyone they touch, including me.

I found my way into the lung cancer community through LUNGevity's extraordinary HOPE Summit in Washington DC for survivors and caregivers, then through their Facebook HOPE Summit Alumni support group, and finally through exploration of the many resources they provide to survivors and caregivers online.

I connected with the Lung Cancer Alliance through their Lung Love Run/Walk in Portland, the first local event where I connected with other survivors. Several of those survivors have become friends. That event got me excited about attending their National Advocacy Summit, where we lobbied Congress together. From there, I learned about the wealth of other resources that they provide to survivors and caregivers.

~

Some of the stories in this book are about other people that have become a part of my journey. If I was able to reach them and get their permission, I used their real names. If not, their names were changed out of respect.

Cover Design by Jennifer Omner, ALL Publications

Published by Basanite Publishing, Portland, OR

DannThrives@gmail.com

First printing, April 2018

Printed in the USA

ISBN 978-0-9996351-0-0

ACKNOWLEDGEMENTS

I want to express my deepest gratitude to my editor, Kate Brubeck, who challenged me to dig deeper and take more risks. I cherish her equally for what she trimmed from the book. The more Kate removed my excesses (!!!), the stronger my voice became. It takes a deft touch to do this without leaving so much as a fingerprint, or a bruised ego, behind.

This book would never have been written if not for the love, support, and encouragement of Genevieve. Her artwork appears in two of the photos, and her angelic visage appears in several more. I also relied on her skill as an occupational therapist to help shape the challenge questions at the end of each chapter.

A big thank you to Heidi von Tagen of Uncommon Muse Photography for several gorgeous photos in this book that are clearly of professional quality. They appear on the dedication page, the chapter on Coping Tools for Living with Fear, Dann's Treatment Timeline, and the author photo on the back cover.

Freeman Ng stepped in under extraordinary circumstances to redesign the book's interior layout. The result is beautifully designed, and pleasing to the eye. He volunteered his services as an in-kind donation to the lung cancer organizations that will receive the profits from this book. I will be forever grateful for his generosity of time and talent.

Finally, I wish to thank my family and friends. Without you, there is no story, because it's all about love.

To Genevieve:

You are my love, my inspiration,
and the most important reason
that I am still alive.

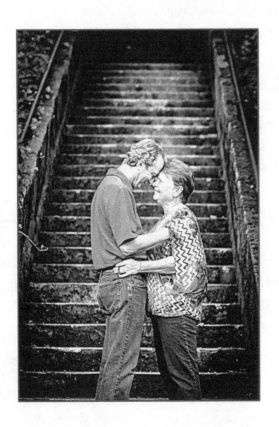

TABLE OF CONTENTS

HOW TO READ THIS BOOK

While I wrote this book primarily for those living with or surviving any type of cancer, I also wrote it with friends, family, and health-care professionals in mind. In fact, even if you have no connection to cancer, you may find that the lessons I have learned apply just as easily to you. Life-threatening situations have a way of galvanizing our thinking and bringing issues of day-to-day living into sharper relief.

The book is organized into four themes: Part I, Attitude, offers some building blocks that have been essential to my surviving, and thriving, with cancer. Part II, Love, Connection, and Communication, is about navigating our relationships as survivors with the people around us. Part III, Taking Action, offers some of the more practical things that we can do for ourselves – some of which have kept me alive. The last section, Part IV, is about Spirituality, Growth, and Acceptance. At least for me, the longer I have dealt with cancer, the more these issues have risen to the top of my priority list.

Since each chapter stands on its own, you may prefer to read a specific chapter when the mood strikes, or when your circumstances change.

Each chapter begins with a quote. The wisdom and inspiration these quotes offer should bring added pleasure to the chapter, and give you a feel for what is to come. I like them so much that sometimes I enjoy skipping the chapters, and just reading the quotes by themselves.

At the end of each chapter, you will find Challenge Exercises which are mostly geared toward survivors, with some directed towards caregivers and others. While these exercises can make the lessons I learned more meaningful, and applicable to your own life, you will still find value in the chapter if you skip them.

Because this book is organized by theme, events that happened during treatment, such as chemo or radiation, may show up in a different order than they occurred. And because the book was written over five years, at one point I may say that something happened "now, seven years after I was diagnosed," while in another I may say that I was diagnosed ten years ago. If you are interested in the chronological sequence of treatments, there is a timeline (actually, there are two) in the back of the book.

PROLOGUE

I was partway through chemo on my second go-around with cancer when I met my niece for lunch. Her office is three blocks from mine in downtown Portland, so we occasionally meet at a nearby bakery. Stephanie is a ray of sunshine, just a few years out of college and enthusiastic about life. Whenever I think of her, I see sparkling eyes and a matching smile. It's just in her nature to be this way, and is one of the things I love about her.

At the time, I had lost all the hair on my head as well as my eyebrows. My skin was cancer-white, and I had been struggling with severe head-cold symptoms for about three months. Due to a depleted immune system, I found it hard to shake even minor bugs. The hardest part of being with anyone during that time was the embarrassment of a constantly runny nose. Still, it was a minor issue in the big picture, and worth the price of admission to remain connected with people I care about.

Between frequent swipes at my nose, I was telling Stephanie about how fortunate I was. Chemo was going well, and I still had two more treatment options available that would likely extend my life. Neither of these options had been available when I had cancer five years earlier, so I was feeling extremely grateful to have any options left.

As she listened, her expression became more and more subdued, until finally a storm cloud rolled across her face. She blurted out an impassioned question: "Don't you ever get tired of being so positive?"

The question stunned me. Was I telling her something so disheartening that even someone as upbeat as Stephanie struggled to see the hope in my situation? Was the way I was thinking that foreign to how other people think? It wasn't work for me to think this way. It was as natural as breathing.

I thought about her reaction often over the next year, trying to gain some perspective. I came to understand that having cancer had changed more than my body. It had changed how I think. My whole perspective on life had shifted, but I had been so distracted with surviving that I had barely noticed. I had grown, not in spite of cancer, but because of it.

Not everyone gets cancer, but we all have something to overcome every day of our lives. So here is the question I have for you: If someone can grow in the face of a life-threatening illness, couldn't there be room for any of us to grow when facing life's everyday problems?

I have found the benefits of a shift in my attitude to be enormous. I don't get caught up in the little things much anymore. I have more appreciation for things that grow, and architecture, and chewing gum, and small acts of kindness, and people. I get more pleasure out of every day. Although I can't deny some moodiness, overall I am more engaged in life. I'm enjoying the ride as if I was just hired to be an adrenaline-fueled test pilot for a new space shuttle. I'm treasuring every new part of this adventure, whether it feels like I'm weightless, lost in space, or in a 3G turn maneuver. Regardless of what kind of experience it happens to be, I'm making the most of it.

I hope you enjoy the ride along with me, as you journey through the story of how I learned to not only survive with lung cancer, but to thrive with it.

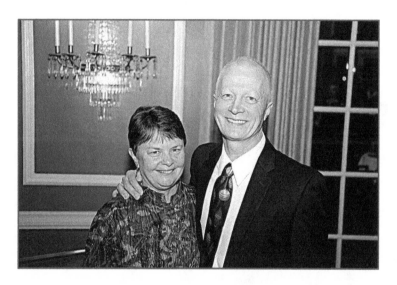

Pale, hairless, and happy:
With Genevieve, at an office Christmas party in 2011

INTRODUCTION

When we are no longer able to change a situation,
we are challenged to change ourselves.

~ Viktor Frankl, *Man's Search for Meaning*

This book is for those of you who have cancer. If you are like me, it will probably be the hardest thing that you will ever experience. There will be times when you will be terrified, confused, depressed, when you will feel completely alone in the world, and when you will be overwhelmed at every turn. If that was the best I could say to you, there would be no point in my writing this book. But there is much, much more ahead, and it can be the richest, most satisfying, awe-inspiring, and life-changing experience you could ever hope for.

I must admit, if someone had said any of this to me in the beginning, I would have wondered what planet they came from. Even to me it sounds ridiculous.

I won't tell you that what you are about to go through is easy. *Nothing* will make it easy. How you respond, though, is entirely up to you. This is one of the many lessons that cancer has taught me:

You have a choice in how you respond.

After living with lung cancer for seven years now, I have

met a lot of people who are facing the same challenge. I've met them in chemo, in the doctor's office, at conferences, on walks, online, and everywhere else.

Since I was diagnosed for the first time in 2006, I have learned so much more than I had ever absorbed while I was getting my master's degree in counseling psychology, or in my twenty-five years of working in mental health. The reason for the steep learning curve is pretty easy to understand. This time, I'm focused entirely on how to cope with this permanently temporary state of being. My life, or at a bare minimum the quality of my life, depends on what I learn.

My antennae are up. I hear the word cancer and everything around me becomes less important until I hear the rest of the story. I have become intensely curious: I want to know who has cancer and how they are handling it. I go to lung-cancer conferences, read blogs, and sometimes contribute to cancer chat rooms.

Beyond that, people around me who know that I have cancer will tell me any cancer story that has impacted their life. They will tell me about their aunt who refused treatment. They will tell me about their third cousin's friend's brother who was just diagnosed. Once in a while, they will tell me about someone who died from the kind of cancer that I have. And occasionally, I get a special kind of joy when someone tells me a heartening survival story. When I am able to listen, I have learned a great deal from the experiences of others.

By default, I have become Cancer Guy. People hear a cancer story and want to tell someone who has been through it. Some of the time I feel too vulnerable to hear about someone else's hardships, so I also had to learn how to tell people that I don't want to hear their story right now.

There are those who see themselves as unable to fight back or alter what looks to them like fate. They get their diagnosis, want to know how long they have to live, and start counting down the days. They see treatment as something that is being done *to* them and that is out of their control. When they feel this way, chemo, radiation, immunotherapy, and surgery are almost impossible to tolerate. Some of them even start wishing it was all over. I am always concerned that they will end up getting what they wished for.

I've also come across some amazing people that have a very different attitude. These are people who recognize that they have a choice, regardless of what is happening in their life. They can choose their treatment team, collaborate on what kind of treatment they need, adjust the timing, and look for what they can do to "make lemonade."

Some want to see how they can start encouraging others, whether it is showing a fighting spirit, or rallying to raise awareness of their disease. They look for the gifts in every situation.

Not least of all, they refuse to accept a diagnosis as a prognosis.

The most jaw-dropping example of this came to me years before I had cancer. One day, I ran into Katie, a cancer counselor that I knew from the hospital where I worked. My job was to coordinate admissions to the psychiatric inpatient unit, and to make outpatient therapy referrals. When these people needed cancer counseling, I referred them to Katie. When Katie ran into people that needed non-cancer mental-health support, she would ask me to refer them to the appropriate specialist. We only had occasional contact, but it was always warm.

On this particular day, we started chatting. Her mood was pretty good, but I was feeling awkward. I had heard that she had just found out that she had cancer herself, and I didn't know what to say to her. She took the lead. "I don't know if you've heard, but I've been diagnosed with cancer." I told her that, yes, I had heard. She went on. "It's Stage IV cancer. It's so spread throughout my body that they don't even know where it started."

This was a real blow. Everything that I thought I knew told me that there is just about no chance of surviving if you have Stage IV. Her cancer sounded even more advanced, if that was possible. If there was such a thing as a Stage V, it would have been hers. Then she said the most amazing, awe-inspiring thing I have ever heard in my life.

"Isn't it a blessing that I've had all these cancer patients to teach me how to deal with it?"

How could she have a cancer that was almost certain to kill her, and talk about the blessings? I knew her too well to believe that she was being anything less than completely honest. And *nobody* could fake feeling as great as she sounded.

I walked away from that conversation absolutely buzzed. *What a rush! If I ever have cancer, that's the kind of attitude that I want to have!* I couldn't stop thinking about her and that amazing attitude for months – and this conversation was one of the first things that I thought of when I was diagnosed with cancer myself.

Katie lived cancer-free for the better part of fifteen years after that. How did she beat a disease against nearly impossible odds for that long?

Attitude, my friend. Attitude is everything.

I'm not going to tell you that you are guaranteed to beat any cancer with attitude. I don't believe it. However, I will tell you that I strongly believe that your chances are better.

This is a book not just about survival, however. It's about much more. Whether you survive this cancer or not, with a great attitude you will find gifts along the way. Gifts beyond anything that you could hope for.

PART I:

ATTITUDE

THE BEGINNING: MY WAR STORY

Our greatest glory is not in never falling,
but in rising every time we fall.

~ Confucius

It was a beautiful summer day, but I was having trouble seeing it. I was on my cell phone, on hold with my doctor's office, waiting to find out if I had it. I had a lung biopsy two days earlier, and my doctor had told me to call his office on Friday before noon to find out if the dark spot on my lung was cancer.

Lung cancer! How could this be? I didn't smoke. I wasn't a coal miner. I wasn't inhaling asbestos. What could I possibly have done to get this?

When I called first thing in the morning, I was shaken to find my doctor wasn't even in on Fridays. I had been calling all morning since then, and I had left several voicemail messages for the nurses, but nobody called back. Each time I called, the secretary would reply with the same words that she must have said a hundred times a day: "No one on the treatment team is available right now. Would you like to leave a message?"

I was terrified. It felt like I had started out one day in a world I understood, but was suddenly in an alternate universe

3

where I tripped and fell over the edge of a skyscraper. It felt like I was instantly and completely out of control, and about to die.

It was 11:45. The clinic would be closing in fifteen minutes, and I couldn't find anyone to talk to me. The minutes were creeping by, getting closer to the start of the weekend. Every muscle in every part of my body clenched, and then clenched even tighter.

Preoccupied with fear, I had just gone two days with almost no sleep.

Learning about my fate was not in the hands of a doctor or even a nurse. No. It was in the hands of someone who spent her working hours transferring telephone calls and sounding pleasant on the phone. One who didn't even know me. One who didn't seem to have any idea how hard this was. And it was *killing* me. Was this gatekeeper who knew nothing about me or my treatment really going to make me wait until Monday to find out if I was going to live or die?

"You don't seem to understand. The doctor told me to call before noon today to find out if I have cancer. Isn't there *somebody* I can talk to? *Anybody?*"

Before I could beg any more, the secretary put me on hold again. I was listening to what was supposed to be soothing music and staring blankly at the waterfall fountain in the park across the street. The "serenity" was such a contrast to what I was going through that it made the tension worse.

Several excruciating minutes later, she got back on the

line. "One of the doctors can review your chart and talk with you. Would you like to hold?"

"Yes, I would be happy to hold. Which doctor is it? How do I reach him if we get cut off?"

"Don't worry. You won't get cut off. Hang on and he'll be right there." Then she was gone, and I was listening to that damn serenity music again. My fingers blanched from gripping the phone.

Minutes (hours!) later, the doctor got on the line. He softened the blow as much as he could: "It's not that bad... from what I can see it doesn't look like it has spread... blah blah... you have cancer."

My body went numb and electric at the same time. While he was still talking, I was thinking about a thousand things at once:

How long do I have to live / what will my funeral be like / what am I going to say to Genevieve / what do I need to wrap up at work before I'm dead / I don't want people to pity me / who will I tell after Genevieve / how can I get back into the office, and get my stuff and get out again before anybody takes one look at me and asks what's wrong and I fall apart / will I be around to see the leaves change next fall / I'm going to lose all my hair...

And more. Much, much more.

The second time I was diagnosed, after nearly five years in remission, was even worse. My doctor called me with the results of my lung biopsy. "I'm afraid I have some very bad news for you. All those little spots on your lungs are cancer.

5

You have Stage IV lung cancer."

I grinned. I had a warm connection with this very likable doctor, so I thought that this must be his joking way of telling me that I had some minor infection that would go away. Before the biopsy, my doctors had told me that cancer was the least likely possibility, because it just didn't look like cancer. So, I had dismissed it.

"I'm very sorry about this. We should get you in to begin treatment right away."

I was stunned. This news was real. I felt a rush of adrenaline that started at my face and flushed through my entire body. I felt weak, and it seemed as if my bowels would evacuate as I stood there in my office. My brain was reeling.

I tried to recover. I babbled that my wife and I had a trip to Hawaii in a month, so I was going to have to look at canceling the trip. He told me that I should go on that trip anyway. "At this point, quality of life might be the most important thing."

That was it. Those were the words that told me that I was going to die. Soon. Nobody had said anything like this to me the first time that I had cancer. This was the "get-your-affairs-in-order-you-don't-have-much-time" speech.

This was not a "you-did-so-well-last-time-that-we-have-hope-that-you-can-beat-it-again" speech. There were no "there-are-always-new-treatments" platitudes. Just: "Pack your bags. You're going on a long, long trip."

I think most people with cancer have a story to share

about how hard it was when they found out. The message may not have been this poorly communicated, but the result is the same. In the end, you hear the words: "You have cancer." No amount of dancing around it can change that.

There's no easy way to absorb the news. What amazes me, however, is that every single part of this roller coaster ride over the past eight years has been better than the part that I just shared with you: getting the news.

How can being told that I have cancer be worse than chemo? How can it be worse than the nausea, and the hair loss, and the lack of energy? Can it even be worse than the "I'm so sorry" pity faces? Worse than the lung surgeries, with those painful, big, fat, hard chest tubes sticking out between my ribs afterwards?

I'll say it again. Every single part of this experience has been better than finding out the bad news. Every single part *combined*. This book is about why. If I'm right, the answers will bring joy to your heart. After all, if you have been diagnosed, you have already been through the worst of it.

CHALLENGE EXERCISES:

1. Write down your own war story. Focus on the "hardest" parts of your story.

2. Challenge yourself to identify thoughts, feelings, actions, or beliefs that seem to surface over and over again.

HOW DID I GET IT?
(AND HOW MUCH CONTROL DO I HAVE?)

You wouldn't abandon ship in a storm just because
you couldn't control the winds.

~ Thomas More, *Utopia*

I felt an overwhelming sense of doom when I was first told that I might have lung cancer. I was going to die, and it was going to be a hard death. My mother had died of pancreatic cancer fifteen years earlier, and the memory of her painful death had never left me. Her death also added a tragic sense of fate to my own circumstances. Could this cancer have been passed on genetically? Was there some bad mojo in my family that was being passed on through generations? Or had I brought this horrible disease on myself?

The last question haunted me. I had smoked off and on for a few years, but I quit when I was twenty-four and have never had another cigarette. Could smoking be catching up with me a quarter of a century later? My overwhelming guilt at this thought was magnified by the sense of doom that came with the diagnosis: Lung cancer is a smoker's disease, and it's going to kill me.

"Could I have caused my own cancer?" I asked my oncologist, as soon as we got past my questions about survival.

9

Her answer lifted an enormous weight off my shoulders.

She dismissed my old smoking history out of hand. She said that, for all practical purposes, I was the equivalent of a non-smoker. "Your history of smoking," she said, "was too short and too long ago to have had anything to do with what is happening to you."

That's when I learned that lung cancer among non-smokers is the sixth leading cause of cancer death in the United States. Who knew?

When I tell people face to face that I have lung cancer, they almost always blurt out questions about whether I am, or used to be, a smoker. It is the only way that they can make sense of it. I have to revisit the question in my mind, and affirm to myself that my old smoking history is irrelevant. Sometimes I tell them that I never smoked, because it is far easier than giving a five-minute explanation that leads to the same conclusion: Smoking had nothing to do with this.

After going through the same disease, the same chemo, and the same fight for survival as people who are smokers, I have much more compassion for them. But I will say more about that in the chapter "The Smoking Question."

Back to my own cancer: My oncologist told me that nothing I had done had caused it, that my mother's pancreatic cancer was unrelated, and that some cancers just come out of nowhere, at least according to what we currently know. Lung cancer can happen as randomly as getting leukemia, or liver cancer, or pancreatic cancer. Cancer happens.

However, attitude, mood, and lifestyle can make a difference. People who are depressed have weak immune systems and get sick more easily. Seniors who live alone but have pets have been found to live longer than their peers because they have some thing or someone to love, and they feel loved in return.

My surgeon is as passionate about attitude as I am. He once told me that he knows before his surgeries which of his patients are more likely to die, based on their attitudes.

All of this makes perfect sense to me. Because I believe this, I also strongly believe that my own attitude is having a major impact on my survival. I think I would be dead right now if I didn't have a positive attitude. This gives me hope, and joy, and strength to fight another day. It makes me feel like I'm winning. The sense of helplessness recedes, and I feel powerful.

Therein lies the paradox. If I think my attitude can have a positive impact on my survival, how can I not blame my attitude for developing cancer in the first place?

Well?

I have been struggling with this dilemma since I was first diagnosed in 2006. I have faced this same question every day. I feel it even more when people close to me make comments about whether I "choose to remain on the planet." Their comment implies that I have complete control. If I do have complete control, my dying will mean that I failed because I didn't want to "stay on this planet" badly enough, or choose clearly enough. It makes dying my fault.

I cannot accept that.

Still struggling with my conscience, I counter that I don't have complete control. If, as humans, we have complete control, why don't we all live forever? Is it because we choose to "leave the planet" or is it because our parts wear out?

My answer lies somewhere between having complete control, and being a helpless victim of this illness with no control:

I can have a strong influence on what happens to my body, but my influence is not limitless.

Regardless of the outcome, the process will have been a success if I'm doing everything within my power to ensure my own survival.

CHALLENGE EXERCISES:

1. List what you believe might have caused your lung cancer.

2. Challenge your own beliefs with the help of your doctor and others that you trust.

3. Whether your own actions had anything to do with your cancer or not, focus on trying to let go of the guilt and forgive yourself. NOBODY deserves cancer.

4. Know that step 3 is a process. Keep notes on how it is going for you, what reactions you have, and what feelings come up.

ADRIAN

You'll never find a better sparring partner than adversity.

~ Golda Meir

The first time I went to chemo, in 2006, I was impressed by the serene setting. The third-floor views overlooking the neighborhood hinted at a nurturing calm that might overcome even the stressful day of IVs, drip bags, and heart monitors ahead. The streets were lined with a mix of tall green Douglas firs and leafy trees showing the first tinges of autumn. For a moment, I could even forget why I was there.

However, the dozens of reclining lounge chairs presented a very different message. They didn't face those windows. Instead, they were squarely facing the nursing station. Even though the two views gave conflicting signals, the ultimate message was clear: You're at risk, and we're going to keep a close eye on you.

The chairs were arranged close together, close enough that it was uncomfortable for family and friends to stick around for any length of time. The confines were so close that it was impossible to ignore the people next to me. It felt a little like going to prison, as if I should ask my neighbor, "So what are you in for?"

I had one of these conversations with a fellow "inmate"

sitting next to me. Adrian was jumpy and nervous-talkative, needing approval from anyone around him. He flirted with the young female nurses at every opportunity. Like seasoned veterans, these nurses smiled and gently fended off his advances. Even though they were close to the same age as Adrian, it was easy to see that each of the nurses had a charitable, almost maternal affection for him. It was also clear that he was a regular here.

Just like me, Adrian was "in" for lung cancer. Unlike me, he was not one to hold back on sharing personal details. With nothing more than a smile for encouragement, he was soon telling me his life story. I quickly learned that the cancer had spread beyond his lungs to other parts of his body as well, including his brain. This had impacted his motor skills, so his doctor had pulled his driver's license. With a passion that seemed to arise in an instant, tears welled up in his eyes. Adrian choked out the words as he told me how desperately he wanted to get better, and that he wanted more than anything to be able to drive again. He seemed to feel as though someone was taunting him, dangling car keys just out of his reach. And yet his arm, his hand, and every one of his fingers remained outstretched, in the hope that he could grab those keys if he just reached a little further.

My heart went out to him. He wasn't asking for much. He simply wanted to drive, to gain some sense of his independence back. He wanted to feel like a man again, and for him, that was tied to driving. I wished I could fix things for him.

The contrast between his desires and what came next whipsawed my emotions. Because I felt compassion for him, and even a need to be protective, I could barely take it in when he brought up the subject of smoking. This comment stunned me:

"The doctor told me I *should* quit smoking, but he didn't tell me I *had* to."

I checked to make sure my mouth wasn't hanging open.

How can you dream about getting your life back, if you are not willing to do everything within your power to make it happen? How can you push the responsibility for your choices and your actions onto someone else, when your life – and everything else that you hold dear – is at stake?

Any mature adult would see the conflict between what Adrian wanted, and what he was willing to do. Sadly, Adrian was not a mature adult. It depressed me to think that, partly as a result of his own actions, it was doubtful he would ever live long enough to find that maturity.

Adrian's response jarred me like a deep whiff of smelling salts. The contrast between Adrian's passionate desires and what he was willing to do to reach his goals helped me to become much clearer about how I was going to approach my own treatment. I decided on the spot to become the anti-Adrian.

I made a conscious decision at that point to do everything within my power to take every step that I could imagine to keep myself healthy.

You can just follow along with doctor's orders and hope it all works out. I strongly believe that doing everything you can to stay alive can be a conscious decision, however. The more consciously you make that decision, the better the chances become that you will make whatever sacrifices are necessary and single-mindedly pursue any steps that could potentially keep you alive longer.

You will also *know* that you have done everything possible, which will give you peace of mind.

CHALLENGE EXERCISES:

1. Make a list of the most important things that you can do to increase your chances of survival. Break down the action steps you can take to succeed.

2. Post your list somewhere (bathroom mirror, refrigerator door) where you will see it several times a day.

3. Be kind to yourself if you aren't doing everything on your list immediately. Learning to thrive with cancer is a process.

FINDING THE GIFTS

A wonderful gift may not be wrapped as you expect.

~ Jonathan Lockwood Huie

How can I tell you, without sounding completely nuts, that I wake up every day loving my life with lung cancer? Even during chemo, life has been pretty wonderful. Not every moment, but most of them.

Every time I went to the infusion room for another round of chemo, I was in a great mood when I walked in the door. I know that sounds odd, when you consider what chemo does to your body.

Chemo's job is to kill off the cancer, but most forms of chemo are still pretty crude tools. Chemo can't discriminate, so it kills off the good cells along with the bad. It attacks everything within reach. Treatment staff have gotten much more sophisticated at administering steroids to manage the nausea, so for most people with cancer, chemo may not feel great, but it takes two or three days to feel any of the more nasty effects. Still, some people walk in with so much dread and fear that they are already thinking about the discomfort that they aren't actually going to feel for a couple more days. For some, they see going to the infusion room as proof that they are moving toward death.

I won't deny that chemo was pretty nasty, but I looked at it differently. To me, chemo was a gift. Yes, it was beating up my body, but that was a small price to pay for extending my life. I was grateful to be living during the only time in history that this treatment is available. I was grateful to have good insurance so that I could afford treatment. And I was grateful that I live in a very privileged part of the world where treatment is even an option. If you can avoid taking those things for granted and step back for a minute, the big picture view from ten thousand feet looks pretty good. The broader your perspective, the easier it is to see how much is working in your favor.

In every twenty-one-day cycle, I would have chemo on a Thursday. With the help of the steroids, I felt great until Saturday afternoon. Then, yes, I would lose all energy, feel nauseous, and get constipated. Chemo kills off the taste buds, so it was hard to find food that I could tolerate. Even water would make me gag. It felt as if I had grown space between my ears. I had no interest in reading or watching television, and no ability to focus. I could stare out the window for hours.

My wife, Genevieve, would come into the room, take one look at my pale, hairless, motionless body, and her brows would furrow. "Are you all right?"

Physically I may have felt like a pile of compost, but I felt just fine about it. I would tell Genevieve not to worry, because I was doing my job. I was healing. Everything was just how it was supposed to be.

I also took charge in the best way I knew how. I exercised. Along with chemo, I was given steroids to combat the nausea. The steroids stay in your system for a couple of days, which is just as long as the chemo drugs remain in your system. After chemo on Thursday, I would golf Saturday mornings for three hours before the steroids wore off, just like clockwork. By the time I would get home, the steroids would have completely worn off, and I would spend the rest of the day and all day Sunday on the sofa. On Monday, I went back to the gym and then worked for half a day before coming home and crashing on the sofa again. I would keep up the exercise every day for the rest of the twenty-one-day cycle. I think the exercise helped with the nausea, and I know it helped with my energy. Further, there is new evidence that exercise makes chemo more effective. Beyond any of those benefits, I was taking control where I could. I wasn't powerless. I was taking charge.

I have gotten much better at taking charge in just about every part of my life since this whole journey began. This growth is very closely tied with learning to make choices in situations where, in the past, I couldn't recognize that there was such an opportunity. Now, almost everything in life looks like a choice.

CHALLENGE EXERCISES:

1. Name five things about treatment for which you could be grateful.

2. Add to this list as new things come to mind.

3. Consider starting a more generalized "Gratitude Journal." Each day, write down one to three things in this journal for which you are grateful, regardless of whether

they are related to treatment. You may want to also include notes about how your attitude begins shifting with this new focus, a gratitude attitude.

HOW TO SUCCEED AT CANCER

There are no facts, only interpretations.

~ Friedrich Nietzsche

I told you in the introduction how Katie, a cancer-counselor colleague, was such an inspiration for me. That's why she was one of the first people that I called when I was diagnosed.

In a fairly brief phone conversation, she said one of the most meaningful things that I have ever heard in relation to cancer. The funny part is that she said it in such an offhand way that I'm sure she had no idea how profound I considered her words to be. "I've worked with many people," she said, "who dealt successfully with cancer. Some of them survived..."

What? You can deal with cancer successfully, even if you don't survive it?

My first instinct had been to believe that the math was pretty simple: Living = success, and death = failure. But when you think about it, those are pretty bad criteria. That would mean that we're all doomed to fail, because none of us will live forever.

Katie's decoupling success from survival was exciting to me. Otherwise, having cancer that was considered terminal meant I was slowly failing. What a defeatist way for anyone to live the last part of life.

I am now free to succeed at living with cancer, rather than to fail if I die from it.

So how do you succeed at living with cancer? The answer may be different for different people, but, for me, one of the answers is this:

Treat cancer as an opportunity for personal growth.

I'm learning new ways to grow every day. I find more things that bring me joy, like tiny wind-up toys, and listening to my granddaughter Lorelei tell me about her favorite teachers. I'm learning more about accepting myself, such as accepting my flaws without being self-critical. My relationships are getting deeper and more satisfying. I keep finding more that leaves me feeling grateful, like the plants and flowers I see when I walk at lunchtime, and coming home in the evening to a warm house on a cold, wet day. It keeps getting easier to find what brings joy, or beauty, or playfulness to my world.

Does that sound more like failure or success? Slow destruction or growth?

Thank you, Katie, for sharing the gift of perspective.

CHALLENGE EXERCISES:

1. List three ways that you are dealing with cancer that make you feel successful:

   a. One that is practical, such as following through with treatment.

   b. One that is about how you communicate with the people who are important to you, such as sharing a successful step, or expressing some hope for how your treatment is going to work.

   c. One that is about how you are coping better emotionally than when you were first diagnosed, such as feeling overwhelmed less often.

2. Challenge yourself to weave these threads into your own success story.

3. Share your story with a friend or loved one.

4. Observe how both you and they react.

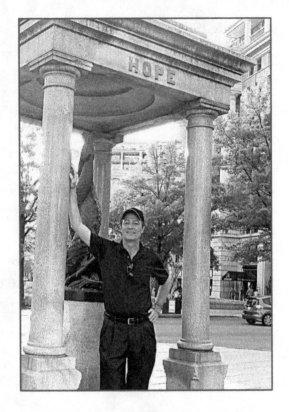

Found it!

CHOICE

I discovered I always have choices,
and sometimes it's only a choice of attitude.

~ Judith M. Knowlton

So often I hear people say, "I didn't have a choice." I find it hard to think of a situation in which I can agree with that statement. To me, *almost everything* is a choice. I want to be careful here, because there are times when people are subject to extreme circumstances, and I don't want to minimize the difficulties of their situations in any way. However, even in a situation in which every alternative may be ugly, looking at even your most extreme challenges through a lens of choice means that you are not trapped, and you are not powerless.

The same is true about cancer treatment. I can choose who I see for treatment. I can choose what kind of treatment I have. I can choose when I start. I can choose how I involve the people I care about in the process. I can choose how I manage my physical conditioning before and after treatment. I can choose to question my treatment providers until they give me answers that I understand. I can choose to get a second opinion. I can choose how my oncologist and I work together on planning the next step in my treatment.

I found that choosing to walk into the chemo treatment room with an upbeat attitude had a ripple effect. The people around me mirrored my attitude. The treatment staff always seemed to be in a good mood. I always enjoyed my interactions with other patients sharing the room with me. These interactions were upbeat, some of them even memorable. Of course, every staff person and patient brought in their own attitudes, but I can't imagine that I would have gotten the same reaction if I had walked in to treatment looking depressed and complaining about how hard everything was.

Plenty of things that went on in the treatment room made me very aware of how much risk is involved in having chemo. For example, there were instructions in the bathroom to put the lid down and flush twice after using the toilet, because even after chemo passes through the body, it is still so toxic that staff didn't want to expose visitors or other chemo patients to someone else's special cocktail. Staff frequently checked my vital signs to make sure the drugs didn't set my heart racing. Whenever someone's chemo drip bag emptied, loud alarms would go off, as if a crash team of doctors and nurses should pile into the room while charging up the cardiac resuscitation paddles. I confess, even if the chemo didn't send my heart racing, sometimes the procedures did.

When all of the preliminaries were done and the nurse would walk into the room with the bag full of IV chemo drugs, I would choose to do it "my way." I would ask permission to delay the process for a minute. I would then hold the bag in my hands, close my eyes, and ask the drug to do its job and kill off the cancer. Next, I would thank it for being available to me.

The nurses would assume I was praying, unless they

asked me about it. While for some people, a prayer might be a better fit, there was a spiritual component to this meditation for me. But more directly, it was a matter of expressing my intentions and my gratitude. On a practical level, there was a positive impact for me in stopping the process long enough to honor my own intentions as to how it was going to work. This is just one way of becoming more directly and actively involved in your own treatment. Intentions are the first step to actions, which then help you move toward your goals.

Gratitude is a reward in its own right. With an attitude of gratitude, the entire process of living with cancer is more positive and growth-oriented. You can be run over by this process, or you can actively choose how you want to deal with it. Your choices will make a big difference in how much support you have, how you feel about treatment, and how well treatment works for you. You can choose to choose. If you don't, then you will passively choose to be victimized. That, too, is a choice. Here is my way of thinking about it:

Whatever you think about, that is what will grow.

Here's an example. You have a loving dog that brings you joy every day. Do you focus on that, or do you focus on the fact that you have to follow your dog around twice a day with a plastic bag and pick up steaming piles of poop? It's a "package" deal. You can love that dog, or you can hate that dog. It all depends on whether you focus on the joy, or focus on the poop.

You've heard the expression "love is blind." It's not blind. It involves selective attention to the desirable qualities while tuning out the parts that aren't our favorites. When two people have been together for a long time, sometimes their focus starts to shift to the qualities in their partner that they don't like. They forget to focus on the qualities that they most appreciate. We say that "the blinders are off," but sometimes the blinders are on even more. They just limit our focus to what drives us crazy, and prevent us from seeing the qualities that led us to fall in love in the first place.

I believe that it's possible to have the blinders off but still have an attitude that helps the love grow. For example, part of why I fell in love with Genevieve was her creative way of looking at life. She sees things in ways that surprise and delight me. She lives in a very animated world. She names her plants and talks to them. When we walk on the beach, she tells me that the waves reach out and touch our feet because they are curious about who is walking on the shore. She takes melted Styrofoam, buttons, and skewer sticks and turns them into a work of art. These things enchant me every time she does them.

However, creative minds don't always follow linear paths. Genevieve is not as methodical as I am. My own attitude makes a big difference here. I could get upset with her for not putting her shoes away, since I regularly trip on them when they are lying randomly around the house – and I do mean randomly. I can't figure out why there would be a pair of shoes in the middle of the kitchen floor. How do they end up halfway up the staircase, in the "trip zone?" Why is one shoe in the bedroom and the other in the living room?

Instead of getting upset, I remind myself that if I were with someone methodical like me, I wouldn't get the benefit of all of Genevieve's wonderful creativity, which brightens every day for me. Whenever the one part starts to bug me, I remind myself that you just don't find methodical artistic people. If I want that creative spirit, I am going to live with some randomness. You don't get one without the other. I've found it much easier to stay in love this way.

It's attitude, my friend.

CHALLENGE EXERCISES:

1. List three situations in which you can make a different choice that would impact your attitude, whether it is cancer-related or other.

2. Test out your new choices.

3. Write down what you did, and how it felt different.

4. Now that you have consciously observed the difference, challenge yourself to identify the attitude you can have that would be most supportive to you.

5. Practice until it becomes a habit, and then keep practicing.

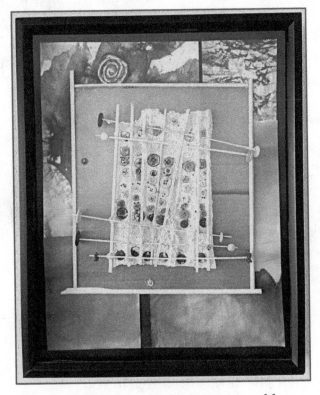

Genevieve brings color into my world,
along with a few buttons.

TREATMENT CHOICES

The best health care plan is a self-care plan.

~ Nina Leavins

In 2006, the first time I went through chemo, there was no doubt in my mind as to how I was going to approach maximizing my chances for survival. Apparently, there was no doubt in my oncologist's mind, either. Dr. Ross told me that there were a couple of routes that we could take. "Do you want to take the milder form of chemo that may not be as successful, or would you rather go for the nuclear option?" I immediately told her I wanted the nuclear option. She responded just as quickly, saying that this was exactly what she had thought I would say. We stayed a well-matched team until she moved out of state a few years later.

Five years after that, in 2011, when I was diagnosed a second time, my new oncologist told me that we could either wait two to three weeks for the results of genetic testing to see if I was eligible for targeted genetic treatment, or we could start immediately with traditional chemo. Traditional chemo meant a "cocktail" (sounds way more fun than it is) of hard-core chemo drugs: four rounds of chemo, three weeks apart; hair loss, nausea, fatigue – the works.

The targeted genetic treatment would have side effects

as well. They included a rash and maybe some mouth sores.

This is a no-brainer, right? Hah! Not so easy! I had a few more questions.

First, would it make any difference to my survival chances if I waited a few weeks to start traditional chemo while we found out if I qualified for the targeted genetic treatment? No difference, Dr. Lopez-Chavez said.

Next, since neither treatment is expected to work indefinitely, was there a difference in my survival chances if I did one treatment before the other? Again, statistics indicated it would make no difference.

So which would you have chosen?

My choice was probably not what a lot of people would have opted for. I chose to start with the traditional chemo, and here's why.

First, rapid advances were being made on the targeted genetic treatment front, so, while there was no difference in the outcome at this point, I wondered if that might change. The cancer was eventually finding a way to work around the targeted genetic treatment, but the latest research was geared towards finding next-generation targeted therapies to combat this. If I used up this targeted genetic treatment option too soon, the "next gen" meds might not be available when I needed them. Having chemo in between these targeted therapies might render the "next gen" option ineffective. This was strictly my opinion, and the oncologist couldn't confirm my suspicions one way or the other.

My second rationale was that I knew from experience that traditional chemo would be hard on my body, but if I did it first, my body would have time to recover and get strong again. My theory has always been that some people with cancer don't survive because their bodies can't take the beating of another treatment. They either aren't healthy enough to accept the next treatment, or they die from the harsh treatment itself. Perhaps, if I got the rough part out of the way first, I would be in better shape to handle whatever came next by the time I "burned off" these two treatment options and needed to try something else.

Finally, I preferred to get the hard part out of the way and not have to think about it, a little like having your Brussels sprouts before dessert.

This do-the-hardest-thing-if-it-gives-you-the-best-chance approach is part of my survivor mentality, and it works for me. Yet I have seen that this isn't the way everyone wants to do it.

I have watched two women who are important to me refuse to take the "nuclear" approach to treatment. Both women decided that the increase in survival odds was not enough to compensate for how bad they might feel over what would be, in their situations, a long course of treatment.

At some level, both were doing the math. For example, "This treatment yields a 5 percent greater chance of survival than the alternative. Based on my age and family genetics, if I didn't have cancer, I could expect to live another twenty years. That means that, based strictly on the odds, this treatment is worth adding the equivalent of one year (5 percent of twenty

33

years) to my life. Yet, I am going to feel sick for the better part of one year because of the treatment itself. That's not a trade-off I'm willing to make."

It may have been far less calculated than that. It may have been as simple as thinking, "The treatment doesn't seem worth it." However, both of these women have remained cancer-free so far, and they are happy with their decisions, so who is to say which way is best?

There are a lot of things to consider when deciding what kind of treatment approach is best for you. Part of this includes understanding what kind of impact your decision has on your loved ones. In both cases, these women did not consult their husbands. These men understood that it wasn't their decision to make: It wasn't their body, so they wouldn't have to put up with the side effects. But knowing that didn't make it any easier; they were both far more concerned about losing their loved ones. My heart goes out to the husbands of these two women. They had no control over what kind of treatment their wives chose, yet they will have to live with the consequences. Their lives may be radically altered by something over which they have no say.

So whose life is it? Yours, of course. Ultimately, you are the one who has to live, or die, with the treatment decisions. The decision has to be yours.

That doesn't mean you can ignore your loved ones, however. The way you choose to involve them in your decisions is very important to them, and to your relationships with them. I don't claim to have the answer, but it is my opinion that, while you should make the decision, they should be able to give you input.

From Genevieve, I have learned that it is very important for me to let her know that I understand her desires, and that I have considered them. I love her, and I want her to go through this process in the best way possible. I also need her support. How could I shut her out of this process on the one hand, and on the other hand expect her to be there for me when I need her? Returning to my first oncologist's question as to whether I wanted to take the nuclear option, I didn't need to have a discussion with Genevieve before answering. I already knew that she and I were on the same page. The subtle drop of her shoulders as she exhaled, her comforting squeeze of my hand, and her words later confirmed this.

The lives of everyone around you are impacted by cancer in an enormous way. You can grow closer to your loved ones by sharing the process with them, or you can grow apart by shutting them out.

This is another time when the choice is yours. How do you want it to go?

CHALLENGE EXERCISES:

1. List the choices that you have already made about your treatment. This includes which choices you made, where, when, and with whom. How did you involve the people closest to you? Make the list as long as you can.

2. Write down any upcoming decisions that you can make about treatment.

3. Challenge yourself to share these upcoming decisions

with your support person or people.

4. Notice how the discussion impacts your thoughts about future decisions AND your relationship with your support person or people.

ROB, PENELOPE, AND HARRY

Sometimes life's Hell. But hey!
Whatever gets the marshmallows toasty.

~ J. Andrew Helt

One summer, in 2013, I had an experience that left its mark on me. As I was riding down in the elevator after leaving the doctor's office to pick up a prescription, someone got on at the next floor. He looked at me. "Dann?"

"Yeah." I couldn't place him, though he looked very familiar.

"Rob, from the Riverplace Athletic Club." Of course. I had seen him almost every day for several years in the gym, but it had been a while now. He looked different.

I wanted to ask him why he was here, but I decided that an elevator with a half-dozen strangers wasn't a good place for that question. I hemmed and hawed until we got out on the ground floor, and then I asked him, "So what brings you here?"

He frowned, looked down, and slowly shook his head. "It's not good. I've had colon cancer." It was all falling into place. He was hard to recognize because his body had changed. He used to have the muscles of a bodybuilder and could lift weights like an NFL linebacker. He had been a rock, but humble. Now, though he still looked healthy, his build was as slight as mine.

I told him that I was there for treatment as well — for lung cancer. He said that he knew this, because I had told him about it at the gym a few years ago.

"I mean that I had it before, but now I have it again. I went almost five years cancer- free."

"I'm sorry to hear that."

"No, no. It's going great. It's been a year and there's still no growth. And when it does start growing, I'll start a targeted genetic treatment that could extend my life for months, or years, or until I die of old age. It couldn't be going better."

Then I asked him the big question. "So how is treatment going for you?"

Still looking at the floor, he shook his head. "I've been cancer-free for two months."

"That's amazing! I'm glad things are going so well!"

He didn't look up. "Well, it's still early."

"But you're off to a great start!"

We chatted for a couple of minutes, and then said our goodbyes. Before we left, he said, "I'm sorry we had to meet under these circumstances."

I was getting used to his frame of mind, but I was still surprised. Here I was thinking that the two of us couldn't be doing any better, given our circumstances, and he was focused on how much could still go wrong.

I left Rob feeling disturbed. I was worried about what would come next for him. He sounded defeated. He was expecting the worst, so I was worried that if he looked hard enough he would find it.

Seeing Rob like this forced me to reexamine my own beliefs. I was left feeling more convinced than ever that I'm on the right path, at least for me. I believe that what we think about is what we grow, at least in our minds, and that our minds impact our bodies. If he is thinking negative thoughts, what can he expect will happen next? Could he have a better outcome if he changed his thinking? I don't know, but I have to believe it is possible. In fact, I'm betting my life on it.

The fancy name for this theory is metaphysics. In my unscientific understanding of metaphysics, our thoughts and feelings affect our cells. How else do you explain that, with the use of yoga, meditation, and biofeedback, we can lower our own heart rate? People can tolerate pain and discomfort better when they listen to music, which is why it's so effective during exercise. We have the same body and the same cells, but with music, we can lift more weight and run more miles. Our mind is focused on the pleasure of the music, not the pain of the exercise.

When we are under stress, we get sick more easily. On the other side of the coin, when we feel good, we heal faster and have a stronger immune system. It's no big stretch to think that I have a better chance of beating cancer if I focus on feeling good and on healing. To me, the real question is how to do those things more effectively.

This is where attitude comes in. I'm not talking about Pollyanna-ish thinking: "A frown is just a smile turned upside down." Positive thinking only works if you can believe it. That doesn't mean it doesn't take work to find it, but I have found that the more I practice, the easier it gets.

My beliefs about attitude were reinforced the last time I went to see my doctor. The cancer had spread to my bones before I started a new treatment two months ago. The treatment is shrinking the cancer, but my bones have become weak and porous in places. I get monthly injections to replace the calcium and strengthen my bones. This is done in the chemo infusion room.

Genevieve and I were directed to a semiprivate room with another couple. Penelope, a thin, pale, bald woman with an infusion line in her chest, and her husband, Harry, welcomed us.

This was Penelope's first treatment after a five-week break. She had become so sick from weekly treatments that the break had been necessary for her body to recover. "I told Harry that five weeks is too long, and I can't wait to get back to treatment," she said. She let out a belly laugh, and Harry did the same. How could they be laughing when she was having toxic chemo drugs pumped into her body and she was going to be weak and nauseous in another two to three days?

Harry told us that a couple of years ago, he had gone

through treatment for colon cancer. His tone was as casual and relaxed as if he was telling us, "The heel of my shoe fell off, so I had to take it in to get it repaired."

It was a four-hour drive over the mountains to bring a weakened Penelope to treatment. "We get to see more of the state this way!" she said with a laugh. Surviving ovarian cancer a second time? "I can't believe I'm still standing," she bellowed. She told us she had a tumor the size of a grapefruit removed. "Why is it always fruit?" That brought out another guffaw from both of them.

We were talking about cancer, but this was the most fun I could remember having at a "party" in a long time. They were genuinely having a good time, and were completely free of any self-pity. They were focused on today, and they were not spending their time worrying about how this treatment would turn out.

Which life would you rather have, one like Rob's, or one like Penelope's and Harry's? My money is on Penelope and Harry and their great attitude. Whether they live longer remains to be seen, but there is no question that they are getting the most out of the life they have.

CHALLENGE EXERCISES:

1. Make a "top ten reasons I feel good about my situation" list. Let humor be your guide.

2. Challenge yourself to share the list with a friend or loved one and ask for feedback to enhance the humor.

3. What effect does the humor have on your attitude?

WHAT KIND OF STORY
DO YOU WANT TO HAVE?

Stories can conquer fear, you know.
They can make the heart bigger.

~ Ben Okri

One of the most life-altering changes in my attitude came as a surprise. I began my time AD (After Diagnosis) feeling like I was in a horror movie. Asking me whether I wanted to go through chemo or die a quick death seemed to me like a choice between being tortured by Freddie Krueger or being cannibalized by Hannibal Lecter.

I'm not sure how my thinking evolved. It may simply have been my survival instincts kicking in, but the change was life-altering. However it happened, at some point early on I stopped focusing on what could go wrong, and started focusing on how I could take charge and make things go right.

How many adventure movies have you seen in which one of the characters has to climb along a narrow window ledge outside a tall building, or cross a rickety footbridge over a canyon? The protagonist is clearly afraid, at which point someone says, "Don't look down!" Of course, the protagonist usually comes within a hair of falling because it is nearly impossible not to look down, even though we know better.

For dramatic effect, a few boards from that bridge might fall into the abyss, or a shoe drops fifty floors from the window ledge. A long moment later, you hear the crash, emphasizing what could happen if the character slips. It all makes for good drama. However, in real life, as in action-adventure movies, "looking down" doesn't make it any easier to survive.

I decided that spending time thinking about how bad things could get would do me about as much good as looking down from that bridge or window ledge. It's easy to be filled with terror, lose your focus, lose your balance, and get in your own way. How is that going to help you?

I know the canyon is there. I don't need to spend time staring down into it. My toe will feel that window ledge. I don't need to pay attention to the fact that I'm five hundred feet from the ground and that the birds flying around have to look up to see me.

What makes more sense in this situation: Focusing on what will help you survive, or focusing on what it will be like if you don't? Thinking about what your next step should be, or thinking about what will happen if you place your foot wrong?

There was a series of books that I used to read with my sons when they were young. In this series, there were decision points where the reader could choose which path to take next. Choosing different paths led to different outcomes.

I no longer think of my life as a horror story. I now think of it like that series of books:

Choose Your Own Adventure.

CHALLENGE EXERCISES:

1. Write down one step that you have taken since being diagnosed when a critical decision had to be made. Include the part about how you looked down. (You know you did!)

2. Describe how it would have turned out differently, or felt different, if you had not looked down – or if you had not looked down as much.

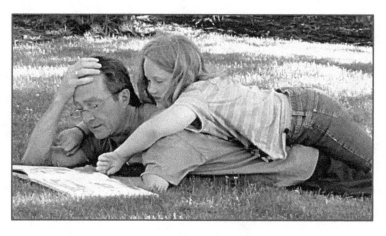

Working on the next adventure with granddaughter Jaidy

RESPONSIBILITY, GUILT, AND CONTROL

The need for control always comes
from someone that has lost it.

~ Shannon L. Alder

It's almost as if my cancer was targeted to teach me lessons. The very issues that have always been hardest for me to deal with are the ones that are the most important for me to learn about in order to grow through this challenge. Your issues may be different from mine, but, whatever they are, I bet they jump out and say hello when it comes time to deal with cancer.

One of those issues for me is control. For most of my life, it was hard for me to know how the world kept turning when I wasn't around to make sure things were done right. The deeper I looked, the more I realized what a challenge this was for me. I tried to keep my mother and father happy before/during/after their divorce, right up until my father drank himself to death. I have barked instructions at Genevieve while she was cutting my hair. The recycling has to be done just right. I have a hard time letting Genevieve drive without coaching her. (To be fair, that one goes both ways.)

For me, the need for control comes from feeling

responsible for everything around me. Since I feel responsible, I have to make sure everything is done right, or it will fall apart.

That's where the other biggie for me comes in: Guilt. If things don't go right, then it's my fault. Everything. Lights left on around the house. Pollution. Global warming. Cancer.

Especially cancer.

Every medical professional that I have talked with or read about has said that nothing I did could have caused it, that this cancer is completely random. The fact that it isn't my fault may be considered medical truth, but it has not stopped me from feeling guilty. If something life-threatening happens to me, it must be my fault, right? How else does the world make any sense? There is cause, and then there is effect. I must have done something.

I have been through every type of mental gymnastics to figure out how I am responsible for something that I could not have caused. Reality was not going to be an obstacle, because not having a cause doesn't fit into *my* version of reality. I have continued running this over in my mind for eight years and counting.

I have faced two challenges in accepting that it's not my fault. One of them I just described: It doesn't fit my version of reality. The other is much more survival oriented, which makes it much harder to let go. Here is the dilemma:

If I didn't cause it, then I can't stop it. If I can't stop it, then I'm going to die.

Would *you* want to let go of control in this situation?

Let's make it just a little bit tougher. When we're under stress, we revert to our oldest, most trusted, most instinctual coping skills. For me, that goes back to control.

Genevieve has unknowingly helped me find a way out of this corner. She has tried to *will* me to health by insisting that I have the ability to cure myself if I want it badly enough. This has left me feeling doubly guilty: 1) if I can cure myself, it means I must have also caused it myself; and 2) if I don't cure myself, it's my fault.

I couldn't find a way to explain to Genevieve why I wanted her to stop telling me this. But because she persisted, she became an excellent devil's advocate. I was backed into a corner, so I fought much harder to get out.

I have finally found an explanation that makes sense to me, and that helps all the pieces fall into place without fault or guilt. I have decided to accept the medical reality that I didn't cause it, and also to accept that I can't cure it. I might, however, be able to have some influence over what happens.

There is a range of possible outcomes, and the place where I end up within the range improves if I make healthy choices. I have been making healthy choices, and I have lived much longer than expected.

The guilt had been eating at me. Accepting this theory lifted an enormous weight. I let go of trying to control something that I couldn't control. And, along with letting go, the feeling of responsibility and guilt melted away. I no longer feel guilty if I don't try the latest anti-cancer diet, stop eating sugar (although I had already cut down), or go to Mexico for the latest breakthrough wonder treatment. This new feeling of freedom lifted my spirits enormously.

Not only that, but there was a huge bonus to letting go of control: I had removed another cancer from my life. For me, that cancer was guilt.

How ironic. It goes completely against my instincts. By letting go of control, I'm taking better care of myself. And I may live longer because of it.

As my surgeon excitedly told me five years after he removed one of my lungs, "It's not often you get to shake the hand of a Stage III lung cancer survivor." That was three years ago. So far, the influence theory is working for me.

CHALLENGE EXERCISES:

1. Write down three things that are related to cancer that you feel guilty about doing or not doing.

2. Of these three things, which of these can you control, which of these can you influence, and which of these are beyond your control or influence?

3. Ask yourself if letting go of what you have no control of lifts any weight off your shoulders.

4. For the items over which you have some influence, decide if you want to act differently. If not, forgive yourself. You have made a conscious choice.

5. Remember, you can always come back to these choices and reconsider.

TRY NOT TO HELP

We are Divine enough to ask
and we are important enough to receive.

~ Wayne Dyer

"Try not to help."

That's what the radiation tech told me while I was on the treatment table. It wasn't a message that sank in easily.

That's probably why she had to tell me three times.

The reason she didn't want me to help was pretty simple. She was trying to align the laser crosshairs shooting down from the ceiling with the three pinpoint tattoos on my hips, so the radiation could hit my body exactly where it needed to go. I couldn't see the laser crosshairs *or* the tattoos. The best way to help was to not help.

This has been one of the hardest lessons for me to learn. I want to do everything all by myself, just like I've always done. I grew up with a father who was alcoholic and a mother who alternated between neglecting me and controlling me. The combination made being fiercely independent the only rational option.

The lesson of this cancer opportunity, cleverly disguised as a problem, is that I can't do this by myself. This has forced me to re-examine a lifetime of being so independent.

Being self-sufficient has been great in many ways. I have taken care of everything I needed to, and on my own schedule.

I have never had to impose on other people, never had to inconvenience them. I have never had to worry about whether they were helping me because they wanted to, or because they felt sorry for me, or because they felt obligated. I have never had to worry about how they felt about me. As a bonus, I have never had to feel indebted or obligated to them.

All of this has also been a problem, however. Being totally self-sufficient has meant being insulated from vulnerability, from having to trust. From having to know how much (or – my fear – how little) people care about me. It has meant almost never having to be connected to another human being. From this vantage point, self-sufficiency starts looking less like a virtue and more like a way of cutting myself off from the world.

This is one of the gifts of cancer. I'm not re-evaluating how I connect with the world because I got a sudden urge to be more introspective. I'm taking a fresh look because this cancer has yanked me off my feet, shaken me up, and spun me around a few times.

At different times during treatment, particularly during chemo, surgery, and radiation, I don't have the energy to help with chores around the house, so I have to let Genevieve do them for me. I haven't always had the energy even to visit with friends. I have had to learn to accept friends and neighbors bringing over meals, and sending cards, and showing random acts of kindness. How self-sufficient can you feel when people call to ask what they can do to help, and you have to admit you need them? How do I ever give them as much as they have given me? It's not possible. I can only express my gratitude and accept their gifts of love.

I can't balance the scales, so I have had to learn that it's not about balancing the scales.

I can't reciprocate the giving, so I have had to learn that the people I care about aren't in it to get something from me.

I can't keep my shields up, so I have had to learn that they love me for who I am, not for the selected parts of me that I think they want to see.

This has been the lesson of a lifetime for me. I have learned that people can care about me and love me for who I am.

Even without my help.

CHALLENGE EXERCISES:

1. List three examples of times when you brushed off help or support that would have made your life a little easier.

2. Write down what would happen if you accepted this help or support next time. How would you feel? How do you think the helper would feel?

3. List a few ways that friends or loved ones could help or support you in the future, so that you are prepared when they ask.

LIFE EXPECTANCY

I do not fear death. I had been dead for
billions and billions of years before I was born,
and had not suffered the slightest inconvenience from it.

~ Mark Twain

It seems as though somewhere around the age of twenty-five or thirty, people stop celebrating their birthdays and start lamenting how old they are. Every year is more of a drag, because they are a year older than they were when they thought they were old *last* year.

I look at it very differently. I am approaching my fifty-seventh birthday, and I plan to celebrate with gusto. Why is my approach so different?

It's pretty easy to figure out. I'm grateful that I am still alive to see another year. Without the miracles of modern medical care, I would have been dead by the age of fifty. Every day is a gift.

I started gaining even more perspective when I saw a National Geographic article about the average lifespan of people in different parts of the world. Here I am, living with a cancer that is usually fatal, and the common reaction of people I know is to consider it tragic that I could die so young. In comparison, however, I have already lived five years longer than the average Nigerian male; I think of myself as way too young to die, but if I had been born in Nigeria, I would be considered blessed to still be alive. I have already lived a year longer than the average South African. We in the West are perhaps blissfully ignorant of the plight of people in other parts of the world.

This National Geographic article inspired me to take a broader view, which gave me an even greater appreciation of my circumstances. For example, let's go beyond simple geography. In the history of humankind, our species has never lived this long. In 1930, the average white male lived to the age of fifty-eight. Prior to that time, I would have been considered fortunate to live to my current relatively ripe old age.

Expanding my thinking even further, I started researching the lifespans of different species. I am proud to say that in two months, I will have outlived the average American Alligator, and I have already outlived the average camel by twenty-seven years.

Closer to home, I have outlived our genetic cousins, the chimpanzees, by thirty-seven years. Take *that*, banana boy!

Still, I haven't lived *close* to the average lifespan of some other animals. But who would want to be a turkey buzzard, even with an average lifespan of 118 years?

Perhaps longevity isn't everything after all. If it was, wouldn't you want to be a Galapagos land tortoise, with an average lifespan of 193 years? They must scoff at us puny humans. Still, how fulfilling would your life be, moving around in sloooow motion? A life like that would probably feel like it lasted a lot longer than 193 years.

This brought me to yet another realization:

The number of years we live is important, but the quality of the years that we have is vastly underrated.

I am grateful for the wonderful life that I have. At the same time, this realization makes me even more committed to making the most of living in the present.

I'm also grateful that I'm not a turkey buzzard.

CHALLENGE EXERCISES:

1. Make a list of what you would still need to do to feel like you have lived a full life.

2. #1 is a trick question! You may already feel like you have lived a full life! If so, lucky you! Describe why you feel this way.

3. If not, do the things on your list that you can, while you still have the opportunity.

4. Start working on acceptance of the things that you may not be able to accomplish.

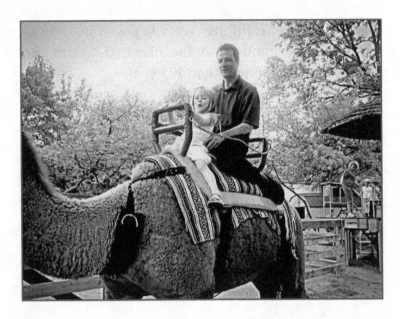

Making the most of my "camel time" with granddaughter Dixie

GRATITUDE

Gratitude is the healthiest of all human emotions.
The more you express gratitude for what you have, the more likely
you will have even more to express gratitude for.

~ Zig Ziglar

Learning to live in a state of gratitude has turned out to be another of the greatest gifts of cancer. You certainly don't need to get cancer to live in gratitude, but I have to say that it has helped me to focus much more clearly on what is important. That focus is a gift in itself.

It is so much easier to find the joy in life once you see each day as a gift rather than an entitlement. I wake up and I'm grateful to still be alive. I touch Genevieve's skin and I'm grateful to share my life with someone that I love so deeply. I breathe in and I'm grateful that I can still get enough oxygen to do so without too much effort. There is a lot to be grateful for, even before I get out of bed.

When people ask me, "How are you?" I usually respond with something like, "I'm great!" or "So far, so excellent!" I don't say this to be falsely cheerful. I say this because that is exactly how I feel. Never mind that I have Stage IV lung cancer. I could be dead right now, but I'm not. Doesn't that make it a pretty great day?

I had a headache that was just short of a migraine that lasted for a year. I'm not talking about every now and then. I'm talking about waking up with a severe headache, having a severe headache all day, and going to bed with a severe headache. Every day. The non-stop headache was an uncommon side effect of a chemo maintenance drug. To attempt to manage the headaches, I was taking jumbo doses of opiates, as well as Tylenol, Motrin, and Aleve. Combined, these meds dulled the pain, left me a little nauseous and constipated, and took away a chunk of my energy.

Despite all of this, I was still excited at how well I was doing. What was more important? Having a headache or stopping cancer in its tracks?

When the headaches started to go away, the improvement came so suddenly that I had withdrawal symptoms from decreasing the opiates so fast. I felt jittery, like my muscles wanted to jump out of my skin. I couldn't sit still. Every now and then I couldn't stand it any longer, so I had to jump up and either sprint several laps around the house, or do push-ups until I was exhausted. At night, I got very little sleep, because I kept leaping out of bed every few minutes.

Was this a reason to feel sorry for myself? Absolutely not. This was a time to celebrate. The headaches were going away, and the withdrawal symptoms were the proof.

So much in life is perspective. For me, it's not a matter of being unrealistically optimistic. If I tried that approach, it would just depress me, because I would know it was a lie. It is instead a matter of finding meaning in the moment, the gifts in the situation, and seeing the big picture.

The great part about living this way is that the more you look for things to be grateful for, the more you find. Try it for a day, or an hour, or even five minutes. You'll see what I mean.

Maybe you'll even be grateful to yourself for strengthening a skill that makes you feel better every time you use it.

CHALLENGE EXERCISES:

1. Think of some part of treatment that is hard for you right now. If none are hard, think of some part that was hard in the past.

2. Consider treatment from several different perspectives. Examples: I'm lucky treatment is available to me; it's better than treatment X that I could have had; or this treatment gave me the best shot.

3. Notice if any of these perspectives bring with them increased gratitude.

4. Yes, write it all down.

5. Thank yourself for caring enough to go through this effort to learn and practice a new skill.

COPING TOOLS FOR LIVING WITH FEAR

This is a wonderful day. I've never seen this one before.

~ Maya Angelou

One of the most useful things that I have learned from cancer has a major impact on my daily life, yet it is something that I have to keep relearning. The concept is not all that hard:

Stay in the present. Enjoy today. Don't worry about tomorrow until tomorrow is here.

The benefits of using this approach are pretty easy to see. If I focus on what typically happens to someone with Stage IV lung cancer, it would be easy to stay curled up in my bed in the dark all day. This is not helpful. This does not feel good. Why would I want to do this? Instead, I can focus on what I am doing right now, which is sitting on the beach in Hawaii. Now doesn't that sound like a whole lot more fun? What would you rather think about: IVs and monitors or sun and waves? Yes, there is a choice. Even if you are not on a beach in Hawaii.

Should you think about the yard work that needs to be done next weekend, or would you rather enjoy looking at how beautiful the garden is right now? Do you want to come home at night and ruminate over a problem at work, or enjoy the company of your loved ones that are in the room with you?

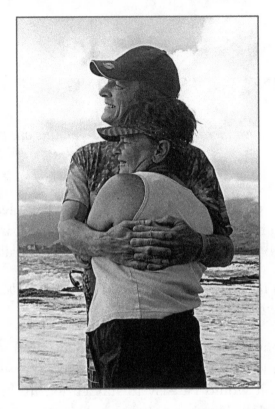

Living in the present with Genevieve? Yes, please.

I can't say I'm a total model citizen in this regard. Sometimes I still have a hard time staying out of my own way in situations that are even moderately challenging. For example, I am a detail person by nature. Give me just about any situation and I'm going to want to know more about it before I make a decision. Once you give me more information, I'll probably have more questions.

When my doctor tells me, "I recommend that we try

treatment X," I naturally want to ask him, "What are the side effects?" But I don't stop there. I want to know, "If I get that side effect, what do we do?" And *then* I want to know, "If that treatment doesn't work, what do we try next? What are the side effects? How do we treat them?" I could follow this spiral to the point of absurdity.

Actually, I do.

If I listen to my rational, live-in-the-present mantra, I stop after the first one or two questions. I don't need to know the rest, and, besides, it only makes me worry. This works great... if I listen.

At this moment, I'm not on any treatment until/unless the cancer grows enough to impact my daily functioning. I know what the next treatment is going to be. It will be a new cancer wonder drug, a genetically targeted therapy in pill form with almost no side effects. That all sounds great, until I go online and start looking for problems.

Did I say problems? I mean side effects.

I guess you find what you are looking for, because it turns out that even the new wonder drug has side effects for some people. Of course, I have to read what they are. Then of course, I start worrying that I might be the one to get them. And so I go on a blog for the wonder drug, and find new things to worry about. *Stop it already.* I have been off all treatment for ten months as I am writing this, and off and on over that time I have wasted time and energy worrying about what is unlikely to ever happen when I go on this new treatment.

The above example was only moderately challenging, yet I still don't find it easy. There are times when the fear is much more acute, completely overwhelming my ability to live in the present. Yet when living in the present fails, there are still other tools you can use.

For example, in the last ten years, I have had about forty-six CT scans of my lungs and abdomen, a PET scan, four MRIs of my brain, and one bone scan of my entire body. Every one of these scans was undertaken to find out if the cancer had grown, shrunk, or remained stable. Every one of these scans told us something about how long I might live. Yes, I was afraid.

In the beginning, the tension would build for Genevieve and me for two or three weeks before each scan, as we feared what the results might be. The scans themselves evoked anxiety. There was the turbo-charged current of air swooshing inside the CT machine to keep it cool, and the WOOH-WOOH-WOOH and high-speed whining as the imaging machinery started spinning around me at increasing speeds. It sounded like it was ready for takeoff. On many of these scans, radioactive contrast die was injected into my veins, bringing with it a warm flush, first to my face, then to my torso, and finally to my arms and legs. All of this reminded me that something big and unimaginably critical was happening. Then there was the two- to four-day wait between the test and the doctor appointment to get the results, the highest anxiety time of all. People call this time "scanxiety" for a reason.

For most of these years, the strategy Genevieve and I have used has been to talk very little about the scans and ignore them for as long as possible. Staying in the present instead of worrying about test results that will come some other day has some real advantages. Why extend the worry? Why take away from living in the moment by thinking about what may or may not happen?

I still have to admit that the fear of death, or of the process of dying, is never far away. There are times when the fear of death overwhelms me. Usually it happens when I'm lying in bed and drifting off. I have no control over what I think about when I am just starting to fall asleep. Random ideas run through my mind, and some of them are about death. But in general, the anxiety has gotten easier over time, and the duration of my anxiety before test results has shortened. That is not because there is less to fear. It is because I have learned other ways to deal with the fear.

There is a difference between bravery and fearlessness. Bravery comes from facing our fears, while fearlessness means that we do not recognize that there is something to fear. Of course I am afraid. My very existence is being challenged by cancer.

However, that doesn't mean I need to live in that fear constantly. I can become fearless for periods of time, and that makes it much easier to have a rich, full life. I can do this just by staying in the present.

Mostly this lessening of my fear, when I choose to face it head-on, has to do with acceptance. This acceptance happens only when I sit with the feelings long enough to take them all in. If I die, I die. I can't control that. However, I can accept that my own passing will be my final experience in this world, and that it will be like none that I have ever had before. I plan to put it off for as long as possible, but when the time comes, I want to treasure it.

Another way I deal with it is to share my fears with others. For example, at one point my breathing became difficult. I shared with family and friends that I was afraid that the cancer was spreading rapidly, and also told them why I thought it could just be my imagination. Sharing these fears took away a lot of their power. The amazing thing is how simple the process is, and at the same time how incredibly well it works.

Ignoring an upcoming scan for as long as possible has been a useful coping strategy, but constantly trying to pretend that everything is fine is quite another matter. If I tried to do this all of the time, it would backfire. The more I told myself that there was no danger, the more I would know it was a lie. That would haunt me, and I would spend my waking hours fighting to hold it back, using up all my energy for a battle that could never be won. I would never have any peace.

I have found that it works better to choose my battles, and to sometimes let the fear in. I have learned that when I do let it in, it doesn't stick around all that long. I let it pass through. That way, instead of haunting me, it pops in, says hello, and then passes right back out again. It comes and goes, as predictably as the tide.

Here's an example. At several points in the past few years the cancer has grown. After getting the news, I might start out thinking about how this cancer will progress: *If it gets worse I might not have enough breath to climb the stairs to my bedroom anymore, so I'll be stuck on one floor of the house, and my world will shrink. I will only be able to see people if they come to visit me in bed...* In this scenario, eventually I imagine that I will die. To cope, I don't block the feelings that come with this thought. I allow myself the fear, the grief, the feelings of helplessness.

Yet to my surprise, allowing myself to imagine the absolute worst is never as bad as the mounting pressure that comes from keeping that fear at bay.

I have learned that feelings aren't permanent. Of course, I had understood this at some level through my training as a therapist, but nothing brings a lesson home like living it. No matter what the emotion, we cannot sustain it – as long as we stop feeding it. By building a wall, we create even greater fear of what is behind it. However, we no longer fear what is behind the wall when we actually see what the scary critter looks like. By allowing in the feelings of fear, helplessness, loss, and so on, their power dissipates, and we soon realize that we can outlast them. We can beat the monster under the bed simply by staring it in the eye.

As a country, the people of the United States were filled with fear about our future when we were in the depths of the Great Depression. In his inaugural presidential speech, Franklin D. Roosevelt said, "The only thing we have to fear is fear itself—nameless, unreasoning, unjustified terror which paralyzes needed efforts to convert retreat into advance." He might have just as easily been talking about cancer.

Returning to my own fear scenario above: once those emotions pass, I often remind myself that for all of us the question is when, not if, we are going to die. No matter how much effort I put into worrying, it won't extend my life. Trying to control the uncontrollable through fear and worry simply doesn't work. So I let go of it.

The benefits of occasionally letting fear in have been pretty great. I have found that I am strong enough to face it, so I don't feel as vulnerable as I did when I tried to pretend it wasn't there. I have more energy, because I'm not spending all my time trying to hold up the wall. And the one benefit that I really didn't expect was this: Acceptance.

I would love to live a lot longer, of course. But if I don't, I've decided that I could be OK with that. In hindsight, I would have done a lot of things differently, but I'm pretty happy with the life I have lived.

CHALLENGE EXERCISES:

1. Stop reading right now, look around, and find something you appreciate. Look at it for a few seconds.

2. I bet that, whatever it was, if you enjoyed it, you weren't worried about what was going to happen tomorrow. You were entirely focused on the present. While the concept is simple, sticking with it is more challenging. When you can pull it off, it makes life less about fear and worry, and more about joy. Remember what this feels like.

3. Think about what you fear the most. Follow that fear to the end. Don't block those feelings. Sit with them until they go away on their own. What did you feel when you allowed yourself to imagine the worst happening? How about after it was over? How long did it last? Write

down what you learned.

4. Share something you fear with a friend or loved one. Write down what it felt like before and after you shared.

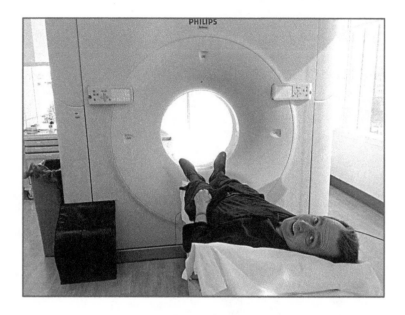

CT scan in 2014

MILK IT!

I enjoy life when things are happening.
I don't care if it's good things or bad things.
That means you're alive. Things are happening.

~ Joan Rivers

In the previous chapter, I shared one of my cancer mantras to avoid living in fear, which is to live in the present. Now let's take it one step further. I found that when I started looking, I discovered things to treasure in those moments that I would have let pass me right by in the past.

The idea of waiting to "start living" after college/after the kids grow up/after the work day is over/after I retire sounds more and more ridiculous, even though that is how I lived much of my life. During the seven plus years that I have been expected to live for just a few months, or at most a couple of years, I stopped believing in putting off happiness.

Waiting until something else happens before you are happy only *looks* like delayed gratification. There is another name for it: "Missed opportunity." If you miss out on the joy of life right now, you are not saving it up for a rainy day. You are letting the pleasure of the moment, which is yours for the taking, vanish forever.

It has gotten to where I now even look forward to

whatever the next treatment experience will be, with the latest one being radiation. I have found things to enjoy about it.

When I came in for radiation treatment the first time, the techs were eager to get me to choose music to listen to while I was on the treatment table. I said I didn't want to listen to music. Why would I want to distract from this once-in-a-lifetime event that few people ever get to experience? I was fascinated by the equipment, by the procedures, and by how the treatment worked on my body.

I wanted to absorb every minute of this novelty. In fact, I had one of the techs take my picture on the table. I wanted to be completely engaged in this moment. I wanted to honor my own journey. I wanted to remember this experience.

I also took pictures from the hospital lobby, looking out over the city. I wanted to remember this first radiation experience that I had shared with my friend, Lorin.

I also got my own private laugh out of it. A few weeks after undergoing radiation to my hips, all the hair in the area that was treated fell out. Yes, that means my pubic hair. But because the template that they used covered the upper corners of my pubic hair, I was left with what looked like two bushy Groucho Marx eyebrows. Genevieve and I laughed for weeks over that one.

This experience was so rich and rewarding once I embraced it that I vowed to make the most of every new phase of treatment. On another visit, I took pictures from inside the CT tunnel, looking through it out to the cityscape beyond. It was a novel and beautiful perspective. I didn't stop there, however. I took the photo and altered it to look like a bunch of cats were actually doing the "CAT" scan. I posted it online, and brought in a copy to give to the CT techs the next time I came in. We all got a laugh out of it.

No one would call chemo fun, but it is an experience like none other. It may not give you a buzz, but it's definitely an altered state of consciousness. It's unique and it's interesting. Having "chemo brain" and growing space between my ears for a few days every few weeks was somewhat of a serene and reflective experience. It's a little like I imagine it would be to take a trip to Mars. How many people would love to do that, would even give up everything they had for the opportunity? Even if there were many hard parts along the journey, it would be amazing.

The many experiences of cancer and cancer treatment are a world of their own. Embrace the journey. It's your own, and very few people will ever experience anything like it. All of the physical changes that come with cancer provide an endless supply of new challenges. For instance, while I was in the hospital after lung surgery, the respiratory therapist had me blow as hard as I could into a tube. How high could I get the little ball inside the gauge to rise? Could I make it go higher the next time? It became a game for me. Then, I started walking laps around the ward. When I left the hospital and got home, I set new challenges: How long would it take me to be able to walk to the end of my street? To the top of my hill?

When I got a little better from the surgery, and while I was finishing chemo, I returned to the gym. I had lost a lot of weight and my muscles had wasted away. Still, I challenged myself to try the bench press. In the beginning, I strained to lift the bar – without any weight. I'm not vain, but I have a little self-respect, and struggling with this puny test of my strength was embarrassing. But then I pulled it together. *Get over yourself,* I thought. *You're doing great so soon after surgery.* I kept working on it and gradually got back to the condition I had been in before treatment. Once I got past the embarrassment, it was a fun challenge to get back to what had been normal for me. Meanwhile, I learned a lesson about accepting myself exactly as I am, and about knowing that I'm doing the best I can.

Every experience in life has something to teach us, but few are so intense and critical to our survival as the ones we go through when we have a life-threatening illness. Our awareness of the potential to learn can be much higher under such dramatic circumstances.

Under normal (non-cancer) circumstances, things generally change less often and in smaller increments, so we may not even notice when a learning opportunity passes us by. We may be too preoccupied with day-to-day living to pay much attention.

Cancer requires our complete attention. If you can see it for the gift that it is, you can milk it for all it's worth.

CHALLENGE EXERCISES:

1. List three interesting experiences you have had since starting treatment. Describe what was interesting about them.

2. Share them with a friend or loved one.

3. The next time a new treatment experience comes up, challenge yourself to make the most of it.

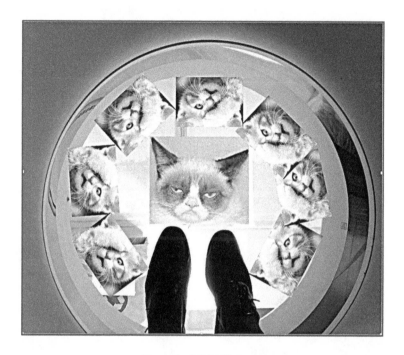

Dann's "CAT" Scan

LIVING IN PARALLEL UNIVERSES

When opportunity comes, it's too late to prepare.

~ John Wooden

I'm living my life in two universes at the same time. First, I'm doing things like clearing out old boxes of belongings that I haven't looked at in the eight years since we moved into our house. I'm making sure that Genevieve knows where she can find all my passwords, and how to change furnace filters, and how to turn off the outside faucets so the pipes won't freeze in the winter. I'm doing things that will make it easier for Genevieve and my other loved ones to carry on if I die. I'm also making a conscious effort to spend time with the people I love while I have the chance, and letting them know that I love them.

The list is much longer. We updated our wills when I was first diagnosed with cancer, and we are about to do it again. Because I left my mental health career behind and now have a second career in commercial real estate, we had been investing in that field, but I have sold off all three of our investment properties. I don't want to leave Genevieve in a situation in which she has to start making stressful decisions about something that she knows little about, cares about even less, and which would have a major impact on her finances. We're swallowing the tax consequences and clearing the decks.

This has the added advantage of eliminating all of our debt. I admit to being somewhat a product of my cultural upbringing, which makes this a very big deal for me. First, being a man, I want to provide for my wife. Never mind that for many of the years we have been married, she has earned more than I have. As a man, I feel better knowing that I have done my best to provide for her. No matter how "enlightened" I want to be about equality of the sexes, my cultural roots run deep.

Next, I grew up in a blue-collar, paycheck-to-paycheck home, where my dad drank up most of those paychecks. Wearing patches on my jeans, I would convince my mom to buy the cheap, bulk cereal that I didn't really like, because I thought it was all we could afford. I also asked her to buy me school clothes that were too big for me, but which I could grow into, again to save money. Being able to pay off the house Genevieve and I live in, and leave her debt-free, is beyond what I ever expected to be able to achieve. It is extraordinarily satisfying.

Completely contradictory to this, I'm doing things to prepare to live for a long, long time. I have been making plans to continue working and to phase into retirement gradually, with the goal of continuing to work some for at least another ten to fifteen years. I am planning to buy an electric car in another three or four years, whenever Tesla releases their "Gen-3" (Genevieve loves that name) model. I'm buying new clothes and computer equipment for work as needed, which is a big step up from a couple of years ago. At that time, it was a major sign of hope for me when I bought new underwear.

So how does this work? How do you both prepare to live

and prepare to die at the same time? Don't you have to pick a path and go down it?

Everyone is going to approach this dilemma differently, and I'm not going to claim that I have *the* answer. I'll just tell you what works for me.

This approach of mine has been a major concern for Genevieve. When I'm making sure that she can take care of things if I die, she worries that I have given up on living. In her way of approaching this, "You set your intentions and you make them happen." It's mind over matter. Manifest your own reality.

When Genevieve and I have these discussions, I remind her that we have an escape plan for getting out of the house in case there is a fire. It doesn't mean that we intend to have a fire, and a fire isn't more likely because we have an escape plan. It just means that we're more likely to get out alive and healthy if a fire does happen. I'm not going to get out of dying if we plan for my possible death, but Genevieve and the rest of my family will have an easier life.

That is part of it. The other part is that by knowing that I have done my best to take care of her, and my other loved ones, I feel better. I don't have unfinished business hanging over my head. That leaves more room for joy instead of worry. Now, *that* part *does* help my chances for survival. When I'm full of joy, my immune system is running in high gear, doing everything it can to kick cancer's butt. Doesn't *that* sound like a victory of mind over matter?

Let's keep it simple for a minute. Even if this approach

didn't increase my chances for survival, it still makes life a lot more fun. Isn't that enough?

So, yes, I can plan to live and plan to die at the same time. By allowing for both possibilities, there is hope for the future, *and* it makes it easier for me to accept either possibility.

CHALLENGE EXERCISES:

1. List three things that you want to achieve in the next ten years.

2. List three things that are important for you to take care of if you only have a year or less to live.

3. Take action on both lists.

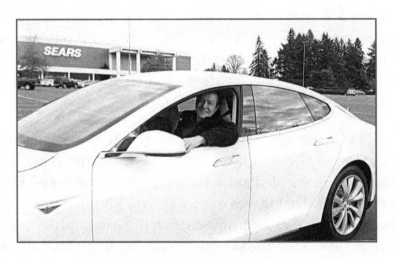

Test-driving a Tesla

GRIEVING

Give sorrow words; the grief that does not speak
whispers the o'er-fraught heart and bids it break.

~ William Shakespeare

Now, eight years after I was first diagnosed, I am writing a different kind of book than I would have written, or could have, after the first year. The book is different because I have become a different person. More to the point, I have had time to deal with the grief that comes with having a life-threatening diagnosis.

In my experience, grief isn't a single loss that comes and goes and gradually gets resolved, the way it would with the loss of a loved one. New phases of grief come when you find that the cancer has grown, or spread, or didn't shrink. Of course, both times I was diagnosed, I was in grief. I was also in grief when I went through chemo the second time, in 2011, and the cancer was unresponsive, because the most basic tool for killing cancer hadn't worked for me. I hit another layer of grief when, due to kidney damage, I had to discontinue my long-term chemo maintenance drug, which was designed not to kill the cancer, but to stop it from growing. It signaled an end to the cancer's stability, even if it hadn't happened yet. When the cancer did start growing and metastasized to my bones, it caused bone pain. Yes, there was more grief. It intensified when the bone pain got worse after starting the next phase of treatment, which (falsely) indicated that the new treatment could be failing.

Grief comes when one treatment fails (three times for me so far) or when you find out that you aren't a fit for another one that is promising, such as when I was incorrectly told that I did not have the right genetic mutation to benefit from targeted therapy. It comes when your doctor leaves the clinic and you have to start again with a new one, which I experienced twice, or when you can no longer go for a walk on the beach, or when you no longer feel attractive. I felt very unattractive at several points due to body changes such as weight loss after chemo and surgery, and growing a pot belly when I was in too much pain to exercise. I became pasty white and bald after chemo, and women seemed to look at me as if I was getting in the way of their view. It felt like a step toward irrelevance – and ultimately – death.

I first learned about Elisabeth Kübler-Ross' groundbreaking book about grief when I was getting my master's degree in counseling psychology. She nailed it in her 1969 book *On Death and Dying*, in which she outlined the following five stages of grief, to which I have added my own examples:

Denial: "I can't have lung cancer! I'm not a smoker!"

Anger: "How could that #@^! doctor tell me to call him to find out if the spot on my lungs is cancer on a day that he's not in the office?"

Bargaining: "If I do things to help other people with lung

cancer, then maybe I can live a little longer..."

Depression: "What does it matter if I go through all that chemo? I'm just going to die anyway."

Acceptance: "Death is just another phase of life that we must all go through. When my time comes, I will be ready to accept that final experience."

Kübler-Ross's work was originally directed exclusively towards loss of life, but was later expanded to include all kinds of loss. The stages can occur in any order, and you can bounce back and forth between them. Of course, you will have many more emotions than these, but these are the ones that have been identified the most consistently among people who are grieving.

This concept is helpful for identifying where you are, so that you don't remain stuck in a stage that doesn't work for you. Think of the stages like notes on a musical scale. If you play them enough times in a different order and with some awareness, you can make some pretty interesting music. Your life is interesting. Your life is rich. But if you play one note over and over for too long, it probably means that you're either stuck or not paying attention. Sounds pretty dull, doesn't it?

Don't worry about getting to the stage of acceptance and running out of things to do. Something new is always coming up that will send you through your own personal melody all over again. I gave a handful of examples of what may come up, but the list is endless.

There is always room for more music in your life.

CHALLENGE EXERCISES:

1. List examples of your experience with each of the five stages of cancer-related grief.

2. Write down in which stage(s) you tend to feel stuck.

3. Talk about this with a friend or loved one.

PAIN IS NOT THE SAME AS SUFFERING

Rain, after all is only rain; it is not bad weather. So also,
pain is only pain; unless we resist it, then it becomes torment.

~ I Ching

For some people, this next part will never, ever make sense. It all depends on what attitude you want to have about cancer, and what attitude you want to have about your life, for that matter. Here is my hard-to-believe statement of the day:

You do not have to suffer just because you have cancer.

This goes so far against the common belief that some explanation is needed. Every melodramatic movie ever made about cancer shows a person in extreme suffering. These movies must be written by people who haven't had cancer.

The view is very different from where I sit. I say this from my own experience, from the experiences of people I know, and from reading chat room comments and the blogs of others in situations similar to mine. The true picture is much more encouraging. A few people complain about how hard it is, but a lot more are interested in straightforward problem-solving ("Anybody have a good way of dealing with this medication side effect?"), and in educating or encouraging others.

My favorites are the people who are less focused on what they are losing, and more focused on what they have. They live in gratitude. It may be that they have outlived their "expiration date," that they get to see their child have one more birthday party, that they are appreciating one last opportunity to talk with the people that they love, or that today is a beautiful day.

They aren't suffering. They are treasuring the moments they have. The pain, the discomfort, the nausea, etc., are real. But suffering, that's something different. Suffering is a choice.

If you can find the meaning in whatever is painful or uncomfortable, it ceases being intolerable and turns into something to embrace.

Ask any athlete:

Q: "Do you have any pain while you are training?"

A: "Yes, of course!"

Q: "Are you suffering?"

A: "Suffering? What do you mean, suffering? I'm training!"

In my first bout with cancer, after I finished four rounds of chemo (twelve weeks), I met with my oncologist. "Not that I love chemo, but would it help if I had just a few more rounds just to make sure we got it all?" (The answer was no.) Although I felt sick and weak much of the time, I never thought of this experience as suffering. It was just a necessary part of healing.

It's all in what you make of it. Sure it hurt when I had one of the lobes of my lungs removed in 2006, and when I had a nearly identical procedure to take sections the size of an orange slice out of all three lobes of my right lung for biopsy in 2011. Does that mean I was suffering? Absolutely not. It only means that it hurt. Bone pain, headaches, rashes, hair loss, fatigue, embarrassing blows to my body image, shortness of breath. I'll take them all again tomorrow if it means staying alive.

And what if you're not going to stay alive, you might be wondering? How do you make sense of it then?

Although each person will answer this question in a different way, the first answer for me is that this is not a black/white, live/die question. After all, we are *all* going to die. It's just a matter of when. If treatments with side effects give me more time, then these treatments are a gift, not a form of punishment. Even if the treatment doesn't work, I have given myself the best possible chance of extending my life. If that has brought on some discomfort, wasn't it worth trying?

Even if my life is not extended by treatment, there is so much to be thankful for. Think about how long humans have been on this planet. Then think about how long pain medication has been available. For all but those who live in the modern era, cancer led to untreatable pain.

Also different than previous eras, treatment has given many of us the gift of time. You may have heard people say something like, "I hope I live a long, healthy life, and then when I'm old, one day just not wake up." This sounds pretty good, except that cancer is the opportunity of a lifetime to re-evaluate life choices, to enrich important relationships, to say goodbye, and to have people we love say goodbye to us. If we check out in our sleep, we miss all this.

Finally, we have the opportunity to find a way to accept everything that has happened in our lives, and even to accept our own impending death. I would much prefer this opportunity to live consciously in this precious and irreplaceable phase of my life.

CHALLENGE EXERCISES:

1. List one or more treatment examples when you felt suffering.

2. Re-evaluate: Was the treatment effective? If so, was the pain worth the gain? If it was not effective, was the discomfort worth it for the chance of a successful outcome?

3. Write down what you have learned from this exercise.

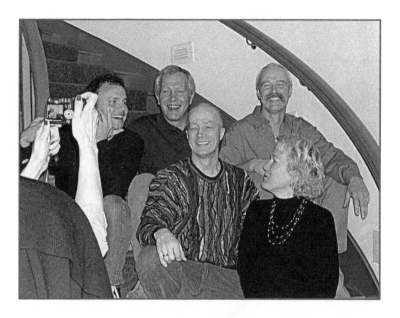

Surrounded by my siblings at Thanksgiving in 2006.
Clockwise from top left: Mike, Matt, Mark, and Dona

WHAT YOU THINK ABOUT GROWS

What we think, we become.

~ Buddha

I have a mantra that guides how I approach cancer, along with how I approach just about everything else. That is probably why you will read this more than one time in this book:

Whatever you think about grows.

What do you want to feed your mind, worry or joy? Fear of death, or love of life?

Imagine that your mind is a field of grass, and you are wearing down paths to different destinations. If there is worry in one corner, let the grass grow so tall you can't find your way there. If there is joy in another corner, travel that path so often that you could find your way there in the dark. If there is love in another corner, don't let that be the path less traveled. It makes all the difference.

When I spent more time than necessary focusing on my survival, the path to worry was a well-worn rut. Now that I spend so little time thinking about that, it takes a lot more to find my way there. I'm too busy thinking about the things in life that I love.

Life is better because of this choice. And, as a bonus, all those endorphins of joy help my body to fight off cancer, and to grow in healthy ways.

I have also used this approach in order to do whatever is within my power to promote self-healing. When I was having a recent biopsy, I was under "conscious sedation." I asked my nurse to read the following statement to me:

"You're going to start shrinking all your tumors and the cancer in your bones right now, and you're not going to stop until it's all gone from every part of your body. Make it happen, Dann! Don't wait for medication to do it! And so it is."

Anthony read that hypnotic suggestion to me three times during the procedure, and I remain extremely grateful that he indulged me, regardless of whether others might think it would work or not. When I returned home, I printed out my affirmation statement, laminated it, and stuck it on my bathroom mirror. I look at it every day.

Will it help? That's hard to know. What I do know, though, is that I am beating down the grass and traveling that path in my mind so often that I am hoping that my body, as well as my mind, accepts it.

If you are going through cancer right now, consider modifying this statement for your own situation, and try it on for size.

Maybe it's a little awkward at first, but it feels pretty good, doesn't it?

CHALLENGE EXERCISES:

1. Draw a field of grass, with a starting point in the center.

2. All around the edges, write down the things that you think about the most.

3. Draw lines to each one, with the thickest lines to the ones you think about the most.

4. Repeat this exercise, only this time, draw the thickness of the lines based on how much you WANT to think about each item.

5. Compare drawings.

STOP THE COUNTDOWN CLOCK

*If you accept the expectations of others, especially negative ones,
then you never will change the outcome.*

~ Michael Jordan

When you hear stories about someone getting cancer, one part of the story often goes like this: "They gave her six months to live." That doesn't happen as often as it used to, and for good reason. The more enlightened doctors do their best *not* to answer that question anymore. If people hear that they have a limited and predictable amount of time left to live, they start the Countdown Clock in their minds. "It's been four months, so now I have two months to live." This is not helpful.

The second time I was diagnosed with cancer (2011), I did an Internet search before my first meeting with my oncologist. I had a desperate need for answers, and I couldn't stop myself. My oncologist wisely started the discussion by asking me what I had already found online. With a dark cloud hanging over my head, I told him that I had read that, for my type of Stage IV lung cancer, the average time of survival after diagnosis was six to eight months.

He proceeded to reel off a number of reasons why those stats didn't apply to me: I was twenty years younger than the "average" person diagnosed with lung cancer. I was otherwise in great health. I had a healthy diet, exercised regularly, and had a good attitude. My tumors might have been countless, but they were all tiny, and easier for the treatments to attack. I had access to lung cancer specialists, so I would get cutting-edge treatment. And finally, I had already beat lung cancer once, so I had a track record. He was giving me the most valuable thing that he could have given me at that point: Hope.

If I had accepted six to eight months as my Expiration Date, I don't think I would be alive today.

As my friend Valerie was walking out the door of her oncologist's office on the day she was diagnosed, her doctor told her, "You'll be lucky to still be alive in five years." Valerie was livid, and rightfully so. She fired this oncologist, and found one with a more optimistic approach. Last fall, we celebrated Valerie's five-year anniversary of being cancer-free, and mock-toasted this doctor. This oncologist had inadvertently motivated Valerie to prove her wrong. Note that the diagnosis was never in question: It is the prognosis that is much more subjective, and subject to change based in part on your actions.

How much effort can you put into survival if you think your efforts won't change anything? How hard would it be to go through treatment if you had no reason to believe it would make a difference?

Now, nearly two years after my 2011 new diagnosis, I have just started a new targeted genetic treatment. I'm working full time, going to the gym every day, trying new things, and making the most of my life.

Would you rather make the most of your life, which very well may extend it? Or would you rather take to your bed and prepare to die?

Don't let anyone start that Countdown Clock for you. Your actions and your attitude can have a big impact on the rest of your life. Whatever remaining time you have has the potential to be more meaningful and rewarding than you can imagine.

CHALLENGE EXERCISES:

1. Write down how long you believe that you are going to live.

2. Consider how you are approaching your treatment, and your life, based on your belief.

3. Write down what you would do differently if you thought that you could influence how long you might live.

4. Take action on what you have written down.

5. Keep adding to #3 over time. New ideas will come up.

ON BEING EXOTIC

A healthy attitude is contagious
but don't wait to catch it from others. Be a carrier.

~ Tom Stoppard

Once you have been diagnosed with cancer, relationships change. You become an exotic being from some alien land, or even some other planet, and most people don't know quite what to do with you.

There are a couple of parts to this. First, people don't *want* to see that they have similarities to you. He has lung cancer... Was he a smoker? Did he grow up with second-hand smoke? Was he eating junk food, drinking heavily, and not exercising? Did it run in his family?

I believe that there are a couple of reasons why these people don't want to perceive you to be like them. For starters, if it happened to you, and you are like them, then it could also happen to them. That thought is terrifying, so they really want to believe that it was something that you did wrong, or that it was something that you inherited, both of which would mean that they won't get it.

The other reason is that if they are like you, if they feel compassion for you, then it hurts them to see you hurt. If they can distance themselves, they don't have to feel the pain. So they try to find a way to not be like you so it doesn't hurt so much.

The next thing that happens is that, for some people, your name changes. For example, to some I was no longer Dann, but rather Poor Dann. There were the accompanying looks of pity, and instead of "hello" they would say, "I'm so sorry."

I learned from this experience the first time around. The second time I was diagnosed, I again notified family and friends via email. However, this time I made it very clear from the beginning that pity was not helpful, and that to me it meant that people had given up on me. I asked for encouragement and support. When I occasionally got pity, I told people to stop. This works, by the way.

I still have cancer, however, so that leaves me in the exotic category. While I am not Poor Dann, I'm not a regular earth guy anymore, either. So what's left?

The only remaining category is "inspiring." Poor Dann, who is hopeless, is doing what he can to survive, and has become Inspiring Dann. The only way that I can become just plain Dann again is if I eventually become cancer-free long enough for people to forget. Maybe then I'll become The Man Formerly Known as Inspiring Dann.

As black and white as those roles are, there really doesn't seem to be much in the way of other choices. Either you're fighting to stay alive, or you're giving up. Either you feel like treatment (with all of the side effects) is being done *to* you, or you feel like you are willing to go through anything to stay alive. You don't consider it a sacrifice; you consider it the trade-off for being able to live for a while longer.

I have always done my best to avoid drawing attention to myself, so I am way out of my comfort zone being Inspiring Dann. Every email that I have sent to family and friends has been accompanied by floods of self-doubt about exposing myself publicly. Each time, I wonder whether people would rather I just get to the point and tell them whether it looks like I'm going to live or die in the near future.

Many people have told me that they forward my emails to people I don't even know. At their urging, I also swallowed hard and set up a blog with a collection of all my emails. Complete strangers are now reading the intimate details of my life that I would have shared only with Genevieve before all this began.

So here's the part I didn't expect: The most inspiring thing that I have done *for myself* has been to share who I am with family and friends, and even strangers. This has taken more courage than anything else that I have ever done. Nothing else comes close, not even beating cancer.

CHALLENGE EXERCISES:

1. List the different ways that your family and friends see you. Do you invite more pity or inspiration?

2. Write down how you would LIKE family and friends to see you.

3. Write down what you could do differently to align with

how you would like to be seen.

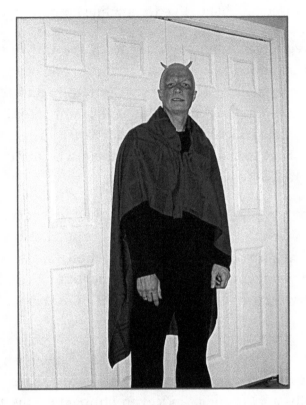

Exposing who I truly am? Now THAT is exotic to me.

GEORGE

*If you can't laugh at yourself, you may be missing
the colossal joke of the century.*

~ Barry Humphries

When I was in my late twenties, the guys where I worked decided to start a basketball team to play in a recreational league. They sent around a sign-up sheet with a place for your name and comments about your skills, information such as, "I played small forward for my high school championship team" or "I like to rebound." I looked down this list and wondered what I could say that would sound good, because I had barely picked up a basketball since high school PE. I wasn't going to look like much of an athlete.

But another guy that I worked with, George, took all the pressure off. In his comment, he wrote, "I'm short, but I'm slow." I laughed so hard I had tears streaming down my cheeks. At the same time, my admiration for George grew. He wasn't afraid to admit to his "shortcomings," and he wasn't afraid to make fun of himself.

What George had done flew in the face of what I believed at the time. I thought that if people saw that I made mistakes, or that I was less than perfect, they wouldn't like me. Yet here George had gone out of his way to point out his flaws.

Because of his ability to poke fun at himself, I liked him more. He became a role model for me, which has helped a great deal in dealing with cancer.

There is no way to get through cancer with your dignity intact. When your hair falls out, your skin blanches to a ghostly white, and you fear for your life, dignity goes out the window. I could say more, but you get the idea. Cancer is humbling.

So how do you deal with it? Do you try to hide it from everyone and pretend that nothing is going on? Or would you rather be like George and let people know that you are human?

You get to choose. Better yet, you get to choose over and over again, in every new situation.

I have found that letting people in and laughing at my own shortcomings has brought me much closer to the people that I care about. Being vulnerable has also brought me support beyond anything that I could have imagined, and from people that I never realized would care about me. For example, I wrote about feeling guilty about the cost of my medical treatment, and how it impacted the cost of insurance for everyone. Several people responded by telling me that this is why we have health insurance, and that rather than begrudging my expensive care, they are grateful that it is available. I would have missed this compassion if I had not confided my guilt.

The other half of the "George approach," doing it with humor, has benefits of its own. The first is that it makes it so much easier for me to accept my own limitations. For example, shortly after I started chemo, I wrote about thinking my hair had started falling out because I saw a hair on my palm. When I put on my reading glasses, it turned out to be a wrinkle. Laughing at my problems is a lot more tolerable than trying to deny that they exist or making excuses for them. It's also a lot more fun. It's a great coping skill.

The other benefit is that it is a lot easier for the people I care about to hear about my troubles when they know that they can laugh along with me rather than pity me. Humor makes it easier for these important people to cope as well.

I mentioned that you get to choose over and over, in every situation. There are many times when I choose not to say anything about cancer. "My name is Dann, and I have cancer" is not a great icebreaker. In situations in which it's relevant, I bring it into the conversation, but my life is about much more than just cancer.

CHALLENGE EXERCISES:

1. Name three of your "shortcomings."

2. Practice exposing your "shortcomings" in a humorous way with a trusted friend or loved one.

3. Observe how they react.

4. What did you learn about yourself? About your friend or loved one?

5. Would you do it again with someone else?

LUCKIEST MAN ALIVE

Luck is believing you're lucky.

~ Tennessee Williams

So many things have conspired to keep me on this planet that it's almost hard for me to grasp. I have got to be the luckiest man alive.

It started with a sore back. At first it wasn't too bad, but over a couple of months it got worse. One day, I went to the driving range to hit a bucket of balls, but when I took a full swing I felt a stabbing pain in my back. I took it as a sign that I was swinging too hard, so I eased up a little. My swing improved when I didn't swing so hard, and the pain receded. The balls started going a little less crooked, so in the end I called it a good day.

It wasn't the end, however. I started getting that stabbing pain whenever I moved wrong. My chiropractor was booked so far in advance that I decided not to schedule the appointment, thinking I would probably feel better by the time I could get in to see her.

One day, I just happened to mention this back pain to my friend Ron at the gym. He told me about a chiropractor that he loved.

Dr. Prideaux treated me for a few sessions, but the pain just wouldn't go away. He told me that if I wasn't better by the following week, I should give him a call. There was no improvement, so I called back. "I think we should get you in for an X-ray. Maybe you have some arthritis in your back, or maybe there's something else going on. I think we should do that before we try any more treatment."

Cursing him under my breath for suggesting that a young buck of a mere forty-nine years of age might have arthritis, I went in for the X-ray. As I finished and walked out of the room, I could see my X-ray on the technician's monitor. She was changing the dials so that the colors went from red to blue and back again as she shifted to get better contrast. It was impressive to see how much technology had advanced from the old black-and-white films. I couldn't make out the images, but from where I was, the colors looked beautiful. I could make out my lungs, but none of the other shapes.

It turns out that one of those other shapes was a spot on my lungs. The spot proved to be cancer.

This was only the beginning of my good luck. Most people don't find out that they have lung cancer until they have symptoms, such as difficulty breathing or a cough that won't go away. By that time, the cancer is usually so advanced that the chances of survival have diminished. I had no symptoms at all, at least none that were related to the cancer.

I didn't find out what was causing the back pain until I had a CT scan before meeting with an oncologist for the first time. She walked into the room while Genevieve and I sat on the edge of our seats, waiting for her verdict, hoping that she could tell from the more precise CT images that I had something other than cancer.

"How did you break those ribs in your back?" she asked.

"What broken ribs?" I was worried about cancer, and she wanted to talk ribs? Apparently, the discussion of cancer was going to be on hold.

She told me that the CT scan showed broken ribs that had healed enough so that they didn't show up on the X-ray. That explained the back pain, the pain that probably saved my life. If I had procrastinated just a little longer, the ribs would have healed a little more, and that back pain would have faded. I never would have seen the chiropractor.

I don't know if my old chiropractor would have suggested the X-ray that saved my life, since she had never suggested an X-ray in the past.

I would never have seen another chiropractor if I had not run into the right friend at the gym, on the right day, at just the right time for the topic of back pain to come up.

A friend who would recommend a chiropractor that I would trust. And a chiropractor who would be just the right chiropractor to suggest an X-ray.

The cancer had to be in the right place so that an X-ray of my ribs would also show my lungs.

The cancer had to be big enough to be easy to find for someone who wasn't looking for it. If the X-ray had come sooner, the cancer might not have shown up, and if the X-ray had been done later, it might have been too late.

When you stack all this up, it is a near miracle that I ever got diagnosed in time. How lucky can one person be? And this is just the beginning.

I had chemo and one lobe of my lung removed. I don't know how I was so fortunate, because even though we caught the cancer before it manifested any symptoms, it was already Stage III. Survival was already against the odds.

The second time I had cancer, I had a surgery to get a tissue biopsy. The surgeon had the sample tested for the two genetic mutations for which there was a targeted genetic treatment. It tested negative for both mutations, meaning the only treatment available would be traditional chemo.

However, I caught another unbelievable break. My oncologist had moved out of state, and I couldn't get her clinic to return phone calls to set up an appointment with another oncologist. That may not sound like good news, but it turned out that way.

We found another oncologist at a different clinic, the Knight Cancer Institute at Oregon Health and Science University. Since this is a research institute, I was tested for all of the thirty-four genetic mutations known at that time to produce lung cancer, even though I had been tested for two of them before. This time, the sample tested positive for the EGFR mutation.

What are the odds that a "false negative" cancer genetic mutation test would need to be retested? This wasn't done at my request or because the doctor wanted to be sure the lab hadn't made a mistake. The only reason I was retested was because I had ended up switching to a different doctor at a different clinic that required a different testing protocol.

I am alive because, after a lab made a mistake and after an oncology clinic support-staff person didn't return my phone calls, I started over somewhere else. Again, *what are the odds?* How lucky can one person be? And yet there's more... but you were probably guessing that by now, weren't you?

Before we got the results of the retesting of the EGFR mutation, my oncologist gave me a choice. I could start traditional chemo right away, or I could wait another two to three weeks until the results were in. I decided to do it the hard way first, a decision that I believe may be one more reason that I am alive.

Even though chemo has changed very little in the last half century other than the management of side effects, "traditional" chemo wasn't exactly the same this time around. A new medication was now used with chemo. The purpose of this med is to keep the cancer from growing, not to shrink it. After "traditional" chemo was done, I remained on this med for seven more months, and there was no growth of the cancer during that time, or for ten months after that. This new drug bought me nineteen more months of life.

I was on the next treatment, a targeted therapy, for almost twice as long as expected. That, in turn, bought me just enough time to get into a clinical trial for the next new, promising, targeted genetic treatment. The trial had only started three months earlier and closed just *three days* after I was accepted. Only 440 people in the world are included in this trial. If my timing had been off by just days, I would have missed the opportunity for this new drug.

Instead, I am still alive at a point when even newer drugs are in clinical trial phases. I feel that if I can just stay on this treatment long enough, the next new treatment to extend my life will be waiting for me.

All of this describes the circumstances as experienced from ground level. When I step back and look at the view from ten thousand feet, I realize that I have even more to be grateful for. With over seven billion people in the world, only a fortunate few live in a country where access to this kind of treatment is possible. Even within those countries, not many have access to world-class treatment centers. Fewer still have good health insurance, which, in our case, has meant that we have not had to choose between bankruptcy and the treatment that is keeping me alive.

I do not take any of this for granted. Every part of it is a gift.

I feel like a frog jumping from lily pad to lily pad, just before the one I am on sinks. If I can stay afloat a little longer, I may get a few more hops in.

Ribbit.

CHALLENGE EXERCISES:

1. List at least three lucky breaks you've received since you have had cancer.

2. If you can't think of three, ask for help from a friend or loved one. These breaks may be hard to find if you aren't used to looking, but they exist.

3. How does focusing on your lucky breaks impact your attitude? Write down what you notice.

BODY IMAGE

You are imperfect, permanently and inevitably flawed.
And you are beautiful.

~ Amy Bloom

I have figured out why teenagers spend so much time looking in the mirror. It's because their bodies are changing rapidly, and they're trying to absorb all of the changes. I know this because I'm in that stage all over again.

It seems to me that I look different every few months. First, it was the surgery scars. I've had two lung surgeries, one on each side, using the "minimally invasive" technique. This means that, for each of the surgeries, the surgeon made a handful of small holes in my back and sides, and one larger hole under my armpit, rather than the old-style single, large, nipple-to-navel cut. Genevieve tells me that the end result is a back that looks like I have been mauled by a bear. I spent months watching the daily progress of the healing incision sites. I'm not sure why I was doing that, since I'm not running around showing people my scars. I guess I'm very lucky that the surgeons used the minimally invasive technique. Otherwise, I would truly be wasting my time gazing at my navel.

Next came chemo. I was prepared for going bald, but I

was fascinated watching my hair come out in clumps. I tried a comb-over when things started getting a little bare up top, but in no time it looked pathetic, so I shaved off the rest.

What I wasn't prepared for was that not only did I lose the hair on my head, but I lost the hair everywhere else as well. Once the eyebrows were gone, I no longer looked like just a bald guy. I might as well have had a big "C" stamped on my forehead. Together with unnaturally pale skin, you can see why I had so much interest in looking in the mirror. How bad do I look? How noticeable is it *today* that I'm in treatment for cancer? Will people start treating me differently now that it's obvious?

Since I have gone to the gym regularly throughout treatment, I had another concern. Losing my hair everywhere meant losing my hair... everywhere. That becomes a lot more noticeable in a locker room with shared showers. Combined with weight loss, I looked like a pale eleven-year-old boy amongst men. It was humbling.

I'm now on a next-generation, targeted genetic treatment. With this treatment, my weight and skin color are all normal, and there is no massive hair loss. But there is a gradual hair loss, with almost no growth of the hair I have. Over the course of months, I'm developing a (more pronounced) receding hairline. I almost want to tell people, "This isn't how my hair normally looks. It's the cancer treatment."

Almost.

In further changes, the cancer spread to a few places in my bones, including both hips. I can still exercise, but I can't run and jump. That means I'm missing out on my daily aerobic basketball activity of chasing my missed shots. The result? I'm growing a pot belly.

One more thing: My hair, which has been curly for my entire life, decided to grow back straight after chemo. It also decided to take a rapid leap toward turning gray. I keep looking to see if the old hair is going to come back, but I think this is it.

So, over a period of just a few months, as I have finished one treatment and started another, the characteristics of my body have morphed back and forth: slim to pot-bellied, dark full head of hair to thinner graying hair, pale skin to normal complexion—and with a growing collection of scars... Sometimes it feels as if I'm walking through a funhouse and looking at myself in the distorted mirrors.

So wherein lies the opportunity?

I'm learning that clothes may not make the man, but they can cover him up pretty well. I'm learning that although one little medication side-effect pimple on my face may look to me like it's the size of a silver dollar, it's barely noticeable to others.

Better yet, I am learning that the important people in my life still love me, no matter what new color and shape I turn up with today.

I'm learning to accept myself, no matter what I look like.

But that won't stop me from looking in the mirror.

CHALLENGE EXERCISES:

1. List any changes in body image you have experienced since being diagnosed.

2. Time for your own "reflection": Write down how you feel about the changes.

3. Write down how friends and loved ones reacted.

4. Forgive those who cannot deal with the changes.

5. Try to find the gratitude for those who can appreciate you just as you are.

6. Write down how it felt to do #4 and #5.

THE SMOKING QUESTION

Giving up smoking is the easiest thing in the world.
I know because I've done it thousands of times.

~ Mark Twain

If you have read this far, then you know how much I value having a healthy lifestyle: Lots of exercise, vegetarian diet, positive attitude, and taking in all the love and support of family and friends.

What most people don't know is that thirty-five years ago, I used to smoke.

Very often, the first knee-jerk response I get to telling someone that I have lung cancer is the stunned question, "Do you smoke?" I usually reply, "No, and the kind of cancer I have is unrelated to smoking. 18 percent of all lung cancers are among people who have never smoked."

I admit that I'm dodging the question. What they really want to know is, "Did you ever smoke?" because, in their minds, lung cancer = smoking.

But telling people would confuse the issue. I learned from my oncologists and pulmonologists that my smoking history had nothing to do with my lung cancer. I came to the same conclusion after years of frequent guilt-fueled Internet searches. My smoking history was too long ago, and too brief (off and on through college), to have been a culprit. As confirmation of what my doctors told me, the specific genetic mutations in my cancer are not associated with smoking.

But so what? Why not tell people that I used to smoke anyway?

I've given you the rational reason, which is that it just confuses the issue, and provides an educational moment. But the much harder reason is emotional.

When I was first diagnosed, I asked myself, "What did I do to deserve this? How did I cause it?" I blamed myself. In my cause-and-effect world, it was the only way I could make sense of it. The guilt was overwhelming. Never mind the facts: If I had cancer, it must be my own fault. Guilt being one of my strong suits to begin with, this time I had it in spades. If I tried to explain that I smoked, but that it had nothing to do with my cancer, I expected people would doubt me... and that's all it would take for me to pile more guilt on myself.

If the natural response is to blame yourself, this must be much harder if smoking really did cause your cancer. This is a burden I wouldn't wish on anyone. Nobody - *nobody* - deserves lung cancer.

It's easier for all of us to give smokers and former-smokers a break when you look at how people start smoking. Using myself as an example, I grew up in a house where both of my parents, and all three of my older siblings, smoked. I tried smoking briefly when I was twelve, but didn't get hooked until college. There, I was hanging out with other students in bars and smoking after night classes, and taking "smoke breaks" with my friends at the restaurant where I worked. All that stuff about role modeling and peer pressure can be seen in action right here.

But there's more. Did you know that our judgment doesn't fully mature until we're well into our twenties? That explains a lot of early-twenties behavior, doesn't it? We are more susceptible to bad judgment, such as mine was (and there are soooo many more examples), before we have fully grown up. Tobacco companies have marketed to teens and young adults (remember Joe Camel?), who get hooked before their judgment matures. How many people do you know that started smoking after the age of twenty-five?

Now, put these two pieces together: Smoking is as addictive as heroin, and we get addicted before we have reliable judgment.

What's so odd is that smoking causes so many other problems, but there isn't the same knee-jerk blaming response when the diagnosis is something other than lung cancer. If someone gets heart disease or has a stroke, can you imagine asking if the person smoked? Would you ask the smoking question if someone had an aneurysm, COPD, or diabetes? How about if they had osteoporosis, rheumatoid arthritis, or cataracts? One of my brothers had a heart attack, which his doctors told him was directly linked to his fifty-year smoking history. Not one person asked him if he smoked.

So let's have some compassion for the smokers and former smokers, whether smoking was the cause of the cancer or not. And if you are the smoker or former smoker, it's time to have some compassion for yourself. Let's do this in the same way as we take it easy on people with heart disease and those who have had strokes. We can, and should, work to prevent all these health problems. Smoking prevention and smoking cessation strategies are critical. So is routine screening of people with smoking histories, so that cancers can be caught when they are far less advanced, and the treatment outcomes are so much more promising.

I have chosen to "out" myself, because of all my new friends with lung cancer. Whether or not they are former smokers, they have suffered through tremendous guilt and shame that should never be a part of dealing with a life-threatening disease. I have heard stories of blunt blaming comments that are at a minimum thoughtless, and at times outright brutal. Isn't having cancer enough, without adding the accusation that it is self-inflicted?

Maria, a friend whose husband, Allen, had lung cancer, told me that the stigma carries on even in death. Allen's primary care doctor wrote on his death certificate that Allen's death was smoking related. When she objected, the doctor told her it was impossible to change. She was so upset that she had Allen's oncologist write a letter explaining that the lung cancer was not smoking related. "I sent the letter to the doctor," she said, "and then I got a new one."

I am fortunate in that I have not had the soul-wrenching experience of so many of my peers. I have been on the receiving end of a few questions that I chalked up to someone simply being too stunned at learning that I have lung cancer to ask a better question than whether I smoke. So, just in case you are ever caught in the situation of learning that someone has lung cancer and want to be sure to offer a supportive response, here are a few options:

"I'm sorry to hear that. How are you handling it?"

"What are the next steps?"

"Do you have people around you to support you?"

"What can I do to help?"

It's time to end the stigma. Let's replace it with a little compassion.

CHALLENGE EXERCISE:

1. In your own words, list three things that you could say if someone tells you that they have lung cancer.

PART II:

LOVE, COMMUNICATION,

AND CONNECTION

MAKING IT EASIER FOR
PEOPLE TO OFFER SUPPORT

You get in life what you have the courage to ask for.

~ Oprah Winfrey

In the beginning, it was difficult to communicate with friends and loved ones in any constructive way, because I was too overwhelmed. When I was first told that an X-ray showed a spot on my lung, the message translated like this: "You are probably going to die a horrible death, and it will happen very, very soon." I was enveloped by a dark cloud of doom and terror. Conversations around me seemed trivial, unreal. I was facing death, and meaningless small talk isolated me even further.

When I felt this hopeless, the dilemma was how to tell people. I knew that I wouldn't be able to handle their reactions if I told them face-to-face that I had cancer. Once I saw the look on their faces, I would crumble. I wouldn't be able to hold back the tears. I needed another way to communicate that wouldn't leave me feeling so raw.

Email turned out to be the ideal way for me to let people know. That way I wouldn't have to see the look in their eyes. I wouldn't have to help *them* to get over the shock. I had enough on my plate. I could organize my thoughts and tell people without getting swallowed up in their reactions.

And they had time to react on their own and compose themselves before reaching out to me. When they did reach out, they were ready to say the kind of supportive things that make it easier for me to get through the struggle.

As I pulled myself together, at least a little bit, through trial and error I stumbled upon an important lesson:

People will take my cues about how to respond.

I have sent out emails that said, "Good news! The cancer has only grown a little! I don't need to start the next phase of treatment yet!" When I did that, people understood that I would appreciate it if they could respond to me in the same way. "That's really great news, Dann! Keep up the great work!"

I sent out another email in which I said, "I met with the doctor and saw the images from my latest CT scan. I was stunned that I could see the growth of the cancer so clearly. It's good news, however, because I still don't have to start treatment yet." The response I got from people was as ambivalent as my own message. While some people responded with "Great news!" others responded with, "So sorry to hear that, Dann."

I may have sent out an ambivalent message, but the response I got was crystal clear. People will respond and react to my tone. If I want uplifting support, I had better let people know it by my own actions.

Here's the next big thing I learned:

The same thing works whether you have cancer or not.

It works whether you are talking about getting a promotion, or looking for a date, or finding a solution to a problem. People will encourage you if you have a realistic, optimistic attitude. When they do, you will have an easier time succeeding. You will believe in yourself more, and you will have more energy to try. You will also have more joy in doing it. The journey becomes more fun.

When people started telling me that they were forwarding my emails to others, this, along with encouraging me to write a book, nudged me into compiling my emails into a blog. Now, each time I send out an email, I also post it on my blog. I also post a link on Facebook for friends who aren't on my email distribution list. They can look if they like, or choose to ignore it. I also post additional content, often photos.

Some bloggers write blog entries, but do not send out emails. The advantage to using only a blog is that you can reach a lot of people without having to maintain any email list. You can also spread your message of hope or education or anything else, to far more people than you know. You will touch, and be touched by, people that you have never met.

Another way of spreading the word is the old-school way, usually called a "telephone tree." You can have a close support person call several people and share the news for you, and those people will each call several other designated people. Depending on the number of people to call, there may be a few levels of people relaying messages, so it needs to be clearly mapped out who calls whom. This is the method our parents and grandparents (OK, and me, too) used before the

Internet. The advantage is that communication is fairly immediate, it is more personal than written messages, and it allows for more sharing of the emotional experience.

However, there is always the risk of the Telephone Game. In this game, you whisper a message to one person, who then whispers it to the next person, until it has been passed on down the line to everyone in the room. The message changes so much from the first person to the last that it becomes unrecognizable. A little bit is lost in translation each time the message is passed. So the telephone tree works best if the message is brief and straightforward.

CHALLENGE EXERCISES:

1. Think of the last time you shared a change in your health with family and friends. How did you deliver the news? How was the news received?

2. If you could have a "do-over," and wanted family and friends to offer you encouragement, write down how you would deliver that message differently.

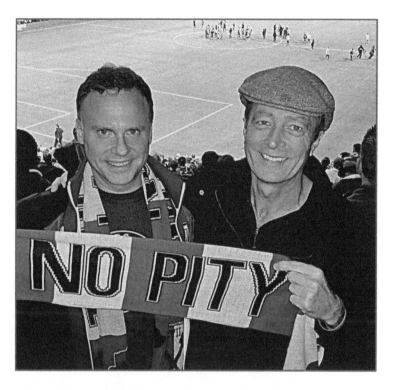

With my brother Mike at a Portland Timbers soccer match.
Although the "No Pity" on the scarf is perfect for my attitude,
it also happens to be a Timbers slogan.

WAYS TO TALK ABOUT CANCER

There is no wisdom like frankness.

~ Benjamin Disraeli

Some people do their best to keep their cancer a secret. A political reporter and co-anchor of the PBS NewsHour, Gwen Ifill, was a shining light of integrity throughout her career, and I admired her greatly. I was both saddened and shocked to learn that, after a brief leave of absence from her television duties in 2016, she died of uterine cancer. I am also saddened that she chose not to disclose her cancer, because I am certain that she would have received a massive public outpouring of love and support during her most challenging time. I can't begin to comprehend what kind of pressures and complications exist for someone in the public eye, but I am just saddened that it couldn't be otherwise.

My approach is quite different. Cancer is a very important part of my existence. If the people around me don't want to talk about it, what does that say about our relationship?

I want cancer to fit into everyday conversation as easily as any other topic. It's not a Big Sensitive Issue. It's just a part of life.

I don't go out of my way to talk about cancer, but I don't avoid it either. Here is a typical conversation for me: "Sorry, I can't meet for lunch on Friday. I'm meeting with my oncologist at 11:30 and I'm not sure what time I'll finish up. How about next Tuesday?" Do this once or twice, and it starts getting easier for others to treat cancer like a part of everyday life.

When people finally dare to brave the topic themselves, I do my best to put them at ease. Why should being asked, "How did you get cancer?" be any different from asking, "How did you break your leg?"

I answer the how-is-your-treatment-going question the same way I would describe a broken-leg repair. "I'll go through four rounds of chemo, three weeks apart" doesn't need to be any harder to say than "they had to put in a metal plate to hold the bone together."

I was talking on the phone the other day with a friend of mine. He was describing setting up his estate. "I want this to work so that if I died tomorrow, my kids could take over and know exactly what to do." After he said it, he got very embarrassed, and then apologized. "I'm so sorry. I never would have said that if I had thought about who I was talking to."

"Don't worry about it," I told him. "This is as easy for me as talking about the weather." I then told him some steps I was taking to set up my own estate.

On the other hand, there are people within the cancer community that sound angry about some of their cancer discussions, and that's understandable. Anger is one of the ways we grieve.

Not so sure about this one? Have you ever lost a loved one and then gotten angry with that person? How about getting angry with yourself for doing something that made your situation worse? Getting angry can make it a little easier to cope with the loss.

Given this, I understand how even phrases such as, "How are you doing?", "You're really lucky," and "Is there anything I can do for you?" make some people angry. Many times I have seen people in online cancer discussion forums express anger, because others with lung cancer have made a point of identifying themselves as non-smokers. The ones who were angry felt that I-am-not-a-smoker comments pointed the finger of guilt at those who did smoke.

As survivors, I think it is helpful to understand where our own anger comes from. That can make it easier to focus the anger on a more direct target, such as new physical limitations, or pain, or, more directly yet, the cancer itself.

It is also helpful to understand the intentions of the person we are getting angry with. In almost every situation I have encountered, insensitive questions appear to have come from well-intentioned people who simply don't know what else to say. I understand how awkward even saying the "C" word is for most people, so I am grateful that they were willing to take that risk.

After all I have experienced, heard, and read, I don't think there is a universal list of things not to say. There are land mines everywhere for someone who is already angry, and for others, there are no land mines at all. When talking to someone with cancer, it is not possible to guess correctly 100 percent of the time. For me, I would much rather have someone make an honest mistake and say the wrong thing than avoid me or the topic altogether.

Although I hate the question, "Did you smoke?" I don't hate the person asking. The question comes from a lack of understanding that there is an implied accusation in the question. Other questions or comments that appear insensitive are almost always based on ignorance, not malice. This is an opportunity to educate rather than agitate.

If understanding alone doesn't help the anger go away, perhaps this example might help: "I know your intentions are good, but every time someone asks me if I smoked, I feel like they are blaming me for doing this to myself."

Sometimes even health care professionals (nurses, lab techs, phlebotomists, etc.) will ask the question. In a neutral tone, I often say, "This is an educational moment for you. That is not a good question to ask. Would you ask a diabetic if they ate too many Snickers bars? You are blaming the victim, and that is not OK." They usually backtrack quickly, and get what they have just done. In this example, I not only stood up for myself; I also stood up for those that will come after me. It actually feels pretty good.

That said, it's not always about me. Someone tried to tell me a story about someone he knew that had died a difficult death from lung cancer. I could see where this was going, so I asked him to stop. He did, but couldn't help himself and told me the story a day or two later anyway. I know he didn't realize that telling me this would leave me distressed. A couple of years later, I discovered that a large part of his family had gone through one kind of cancer or another, and this consumed a lot of his thoughts. How could I hold that against him? He needed to share his experience with someone who understood what it meant to him.

CHALLENGE EXERCISES:

1. List the questions that people ask, or things that they say to you, about cancer that "push your buttons," or bother you.

2. Write down what it is about their questions or comments that strikes a nerve.

3. Practice an assertive response to their questions or comments using this format: "When people ask me/tell me _____, I feel like _____, and I would appreciate it if you would _____. "

4. Role-play with a friend or loved one until it becomes more comfortable.

HOW ARE YOU?

Someone asked someone who was about my age: How are you?
The answer was, Fine. If you don't ask for details.

~ Katharine Hepburn

"How are you?" seems like such a simple question, but it is one of the most confusing questions that I have been asked since I got cancer. What do people mean by it? Are they asking me a general question, in the same cursory way that they would ask the cashier at the grocery store? Are they asking for details about my health?

Even if I know which way people are asking the question, I have to decide how I want to answer it. If I bump into them at Starbucks and there are a couple of dozen strangers around, I may not want to start up a conversation about cancer. If they have braced themselves to hear whatever the news could be, but I'm on my way out the door to an appointment, it may be hard to give them a satisfactory answer. If they are asking the question in the same way that someone might say, "Nice day, isn't it?" but I misread the signals and give them a medical update, I'm going to feel pretty foolish.

This last one gets particularly tricky in work circles. Word may have traveled to some people but not to others. There are people that I run into a few times a year; I may not have told them, but someone else may have passed the word. I have to try to read into their expression what they know and what they are asking. I also forget who I have told, which can make it confusing for some people when they get a generic response to a personal question.

If they are asking because they truly want to know how I am, the next thing I need to decide is how much of an answer they want to hear. For some people, if I say, "The cancer is still there, and it isn't growing right now," they have heard everything they want to know. Others are really asking about the latest CT scan and the implications these test results have for metastasis, if my kidneys are doing well enough to be able to start the next phase of treatment when the time comes, and so on.

The other way of asking, when people are really saying, "How are you handling it?" requires that I again tease out what they are looking for. They could be satisfied if I say, "Keeping up a great attitude!" However, they might also be wanting to find out, "How are you handling the not knowing what will come next? How do you keep going to work every day? What are you doing to take care of yourself? How is Genevieve doing with all this?"

I think sometimes people ask the question in a vague way because they aren't sure whether it's OK to ask – or whether they really want to ask – questions that are so personal in nature. If I had my wish, they would be as clear as possible about what they are asking so that I don't have to guess.

My other wish would be to have them ask themselves:

"Would I want someone to ask me this question if I was in their shoes?" Better yet: "Would I want this person to ask me this same question if I was right here in the grocery store (or wherever else they happen to be) right now?"

CHALLENGE EXERCISES:

1. List three instances when people have asked you about how you are doing that have been unclear or awkward.

2. Write down options for how you can respond the next time the question comes up.

3. Practice with a friend or loved one.

THIS IS YOUR CHANCE

Either this wallpaper goes, or I do.

~ Oscar Wilde's last words

I have stumbled onto something important that I didn't fully comprehend until I had been wrestling with cancer for a few years.

When you are in a potentially life-threatening situation, other people are much more interested in what you think and how you are going to act than they have ever been before.

I'm not saying that friends and family weren't interested in what I had to say before all this started, or that I wasn't interested in what they had to say. But things are different now that I have cancer. People are watching and listening as if everything I do or say is somehow more significant because it may be one of the last things I do. For this reason, how we communicate with the people we love and care about is important at this critical time. They will be paying very close attention. Our words and actions may even change their lives.

Even in situations that seem to be trivial, the same principle – that your words and actions will carry greater impact at this time – applies to everything you do. People will be watching how you respond.

Still going out to the movies occasionally? People will see that you are engaged in life. Buying new clothes, even though you may not get a chance to wear them out? Your actions will probably be interpreted to mean that you still have hope.

On the other hand, if you choose to complain about how hard living with cancer is, that will be your final legacy. If you become bitter, that is what they will remember about you. If you act like a victim, they may just follow your lead and both treat you that way and be more willing to accept being victims in their own lives.

Is that what you want?

You can consciously send a very different message. If you let people you love know how much they mean to you, this will stick with them for the rest of their lives. If you remind people that they have choices in every situation, they are more likely to continue looking for opportunities to make choices. If you show people that you are living every moment and relishing the present, they will take your lead and make a serious effort to do the same.

In short, you have the ability to influence people's lives for the better. What are you going to do with this opportunity?

This honesty isn't just for other people's benefit, however. I also discovered a more selfish motivation. Once I had cancer, I needed my friends and loved ones far more than I ever had. If I was going to have their support, truly have their support, I needed to be honest. I couldn't put on a brave front and ignore how afraid and vulnerable I felt. How could they support me if I told them that everything was just fine? And how could I be an inspiration or a role model for them if I wasn't telling them the truth about how hard it was?

These circumstances converged to help me realize that the best approach that I could take would be to share the hard times, but also to share what kept me going. I often tell the people around me how much they mean to me and that they are keeping me alive with their support. They are a critical part of my survival, and it is important to me that they know it. I have shared my optimism, and I have shared my fears.

Having cancer has pushed me into choosing to become the best version of myself that I can be, because I need that version to survive. And even if I don't survive this cancer, I need these people to help me make the most of the time I have left.

I know I am accountable to all of these people whom I have opened myself up to. For example, after I told people I was working out at the gym every day, I knew that at any moment they could ask me if I was still doing it. It's very hard to slack when people are cheering you on for working so hard to survive. I have chosen to become more open and honest not only to keep myself accountable to others, but also because for the first time in my life I am confident that I have something to offer them.

Sharing anything about myself, let alone something that left me vulnerable, used to be out of my comfort zone. Not surprisingly, the first emails that I sent out to family and friends were pretty much straight medical reports that didn't reveal anything about how I was dealing with the situation.

For example:

On Wednesday afternoon I will have an outpatient bronchoscope, where a narrow flexible cable with a camera and a pincher on the end will be guided into my lung. A sample of the mass will be taken for a biopsy. By Friday we should have results of the biopsy...

The friends and family that I emailed surprised me with how much support they offered, since I had doubted that people cared very much. Gradually, even though it was extremely uncomfortable to stick my neck out, I started adding in more personality and opinions. Because I was continually rewarded with their encouragement for doing so, I gradually took increasing risks. Here's a night-and-day example of how my openness evolved:

First, about the hair. Gone. Pffft. It started falling out, so I asked Genevieve to shave my head completely. Since I was leaving a trail of hair that Hansel and Gretel could follow, she agreed. My apologies to the guys in the office who sit behind me, who probably wish they were wearing sunglasses to cope with the glare off my glow-in-the-dark, never-seen-daylight white head. We had some sun last weekend at Eagle Crest, so now baldness looks a little more like a fashion statement and a little less like a cancer patient. I'm a lot less self-conscious now that I'm not wearing a neon sign that says, "Ask me about cancer." I can choose who I tell! And the good part, as I told Genevieve, is that hair falling out is a sign that the chemo is doing its job..."

That encouragement kept pouring in, and is leading me to continue sticking my neck out a little further all the time, such as by sharing my cancer story at (gasp!) public speaking engagements, and being interviewed by the local television station for Lung Cancer Awareness Month. I can't say that it has gotten easier. The best I can say is that I have gotten more used to being uncomfortable.

Discomfort aside, the rewards for such honesty have been very gratifying. My heart swelled when I showed my fourteen-year-old granddaughter Caitlin part of my blog, and a month later she told me what an inspiration I am for her. Friends have told me that they have changed how they look at parts of their life because they have been inspired by my journey. Some of the people that I thought would delete my emails before even opening them approached me at different times to tell me how much they were moved by what I had written. Several people have told me that, after reading my emails, they told themselves to "get over yourself," because they had a different perspective after reading what I was going through. One family member told me that she began writing a "gratitude journal," and now starts every day by writing down ten things that she is grateful for.

I don't think that responses like this happen because I'm an extra lovable guy or because of how I write. I think these things happen because, when I touch people's hearts with the truth, it affects them in ways I cannot imagine. It's not only healing for me, it's healing for them.

What more could we hope for in this world than to have a healthy influence on the people we love, and for them to do the same for us?

Again, this isn't happening because I put on a brave front and tell them that I'm not afraid of anything. It's because

I tell them that I *am* afraid, and that I am facing it anyway. And then I tell them how I am facing it. I can't say what that communication will look like if or when my health deteriorates again, but for now this personal honesty business is both alien to me, and also the best version of myself that I know how to be.

I really understood the full value of openness and honesty during this powerful time, not through my own sharing, but when someone I loved did the same for me.

When I was thirty-four, my mother was diagnosed with pancreatic cancer. Our relationship had been strained for over a decade, but my world changed after she was diagnosed. She was so honest with me during that time that I was able to heal in ways that I never thought I could.

The reasons for the strain in our relationship were clear to me. When I was a small child, she used to tie me to the garage door so that she wouldn't have to watch me, while making sure that I wouldn't run out into the street. She watched all of my older brothers' Little League baseball games, but when I was finally old enough to play, she moved over to the other field to watch the older boys play. She told me that watching the little kids (me) play was too boring.

Growing up, she provided a confusing mix of wanting to know my every intimate thought so that she could advise me about what I "might want to do" about any and all life decisions, and ignoring my practical and emotional needs. For example, when I was fourteen, she might ask about what I said to my girlfriend on the phone, then pick the conversation apart and suggest how I might talk about certain things differently. I couldn't get her to back off without hurting her deeply. Yet I have no memories of her ever helping with my homework, even in grade school. She never attended any of my high school gymnastics or tennis competitions. My role was to have an unhealthy intimacy with her in order to satisfy her needs, while she neglected mine. It's no wonder that sharing who I am with others is difficult. When I did this as a child, it led to inappropriate closeness and to caretaking of my mother, in return for which I was left empty.

Though the seeds of the strain in our relationship were planted in my childhood, they didn't come to fruition until my early twenties. That's when I told my mother that I wasn't going to share my intimate thoughts with her any more. She couldn't comprehend why, and she was devastated. It worsened when I married a woman she didn't like, and deteriorated even further after my now ex-wife and I adopted our sons.

My mother and I hadn't been able to figure out healthy boundaries with each other. Yet despite all this history, it only took a few words from my mother in her hospital bed to change my life forever: "I'm sorry that I wasn't a better mother to you."

The wall between us dissolved. Forgiveness poured in. The tension and a lifetime of issues were set aside in a moment. For the first time, I felt she understood. I felt whole. I felt closer to her, this time in a healthy way.

In time, thinking about those near-final words led me beyond forgiveness, to understanding the forces in her life that had formed her into who she had become. She became the primary caregiver for her two younger brothers when she was ten years old, while her mother worked one job and her alcoholic father worked two. She left home at nineteen, married an alcoholic, and had four kids by the age of twenty-three. No wonder she didn't have more to give, and that she didn't know how to relate other than by telling me what I "might want to do" at every opportunity.

These ten words also opened the door to a better understanding of my own problems with intimacy, which is making it easier for me to make conscious efforts to grow past them.

If my mother had not been dying, she never would have taken the risk of talking about what was so critically important to her. Even if she had somehow found the courage to have that conversation without the urgency of time, I am fairly certain the power of her words would not have hit me in the same way.

If you doubt that the people around you are tuned in to you differently than before your diagnosis, it may be time to reconsider. This is an opportunity that you don't want to overlook.

CHALLENGE EXERCISES:

1. List the most important people in your life. They may or may not be people that you see often, or even that you get along with.

2. Write down what you would say to each of them if you could have just one final conversation.

3. You know what comes next.

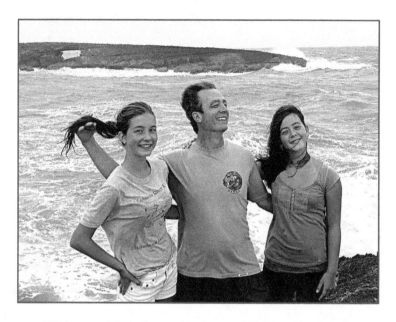

With granddaughters Caitlin and Lorelei in Hawaii

LETTING PEOPLE IN

Courage starts with showing up and letting ourselves be seen.

~ Brené Brown

As you may have guessed from my story about my mother in the previous chapter, trusting that people care about me has been a lifetime struggle. When I tried to give love, I usually ended up drained. I had a father who treated me with indifference at best and then drank himself to death, despite my efforts to get him to stop. I had family members who would never be close to me the way I wanted to be close to them, even though I tried over and over. I had an old history of one-sided friendships.

Years of therapy helped me to stop going where I wasn't wanted, but it was still hard for me to figure out how to be close to people who didn't suck the life out of me. It was clearly my own issue. I don't blame the people around me. However, knowing that it was my own issue didn't make it go away. It has been baffling at times.

I have always had difficulty asking anyone to do anything for me. It is uncomfortable to ask Genevieve to get me a cup of coffee, even when she is already in the kitchen. It has been a major challenge just to let anyone do something for me without my asking. That makes the question "Is there anything I can do for you?" an awkward one for me. You are asking me to ask you for something. Even if there was something that I could think of, it would be too awkward for me to say the words. Asking cuts away at my sense of independence, and makes me feel weak and vulnerable. It's embarrassing.

Once you begin questioning that other people care, it's self-perpetuating. If I don't expect people to care, then when they act in a caring way I wonder if they really mean it. Maybe they have other motives. Maybe they aren't really being nice, it just looks that way. I have become a master at brushing off caring and compliments. It doesn't take too long for people to get the hint and stop trying.

When you look at life through this distorted kind of lens, very little light gets in. That makes it even harder to believe it's real the next time someone acts with kindness. It's hard to look for acceptance when you're expecting rejection. Repeat this a few thousand times and it becomes ingrained. Not only that, but this deeply ingrained habit led me to believe that I didn't deserve other people's kindness, which made me doubt them even more.

I have always tried to make fresh mistakes rather than to make the same stale ones over and over, but with my resistance to accepting the care of others, I beat my head against the wall so many times that you would think I was a woodpecker.

This is one of the surprising ways that cancer has helped me, though in the beginning I questioned even small acts of kindness. Even in those moments, I felt that I should reciprocate. It could be as simple as someone saying, "I'm thinking of you." Really? Someone would do that for me? Shouldn't I be doing something in return? Can I accept having someone care about me? Do I deserve it?

It has been hard to comprehend that these people truly care.

Yet people go beyond just hoping that things will go well for me. In so many ways beyond asking what they can do, they tell me that they want me to live. My cousin Kevin came by with his son to give me a two-inch wind-up robot. Friends call just to check in from time to time. Genevieve's sister Christine sent me a colored egg with a goofy face and wild long hair, as a reminder to grow my hair back after chemo: now I use it as an ornament on our Christmas tree every year. Work friends pull me aside now and then just to ask how I'm doing. When I asked for images of hope, dozens of people sent pictures to me. One friend, who insisted on complete anonymity, surprised me by sending a check to pay for one of our flights to San Diego for my clinical trial, even though he knew we didn't need the money. Lee, a friend from high school, has been riding his bike twelve miles to work every day for the past two years, rain or shine, in honor of me. My friend Buck shaved his head bald as a show of support when I was going through chemo. As hard as it is for me to take in, these actions, along with the cards, and phone calls, and visits, are the ways that they tell me that they care, and that they love me.

Caring at that level of intensity is really hard to miss, even for someone as deft at dodging the message as I have been. It busts right through all my trust barriers. It feels really

157

good. But it feels very awkward. I'm not used to gracefully accepting the message.

After a lifetime of feeling that I didn't deserve it, it has taken a battering ram of caring from friends and family to help me realize that I have more value to this world than I had ever let myself believe. The more I let in the love from others, the easier it becomes to feel that I deserve it. This includes deserving to be loved by myself as well as by others.

Initially, when people sent me love and support, it was all I could do to say "thank you." In fact, the first time I had cancer, I often didn't have the energy to respond to support. Sometimes this was due to weakness from chemo or surgery; often it was because it was too emotionally taxing to respond because of how awkward it was to take in the caring.

The second time around, I rethought this. I asked myself how I could count on support from family and friends if I didn't acknowledge these gifts. I made a real effort to respond, and it changed everything.

It changed for a lot of reasons. I stopped feeling guilty when I started returning the communication, because I could feel the love going both ways. Then, it got easier to say supportive and loving things back to these people. The taboo against allowing people to see who I am and how I feel had been lifted in a big way. It felt great. And, it also *gave* me more energy. Accepting their love and sending them mine was opening my heart. I was healing from the heart out.

The more I healed, the better I felt, and the easier it got to say how I felt. My messages of support and love to others got stronger, and my heart swelled. Sometimes when the people I care about responded to me, I asked more about how their lives were going. I wasn't worried any more about getting swallowed up in their problems or having them "suck the life out of me," because these people had already shown me that they had the ability to give. I could trust the balance, something I hadn't known how to do before.

Genevieve calls this "changing your vibration." I call it learning how to love. Either way, if you can do this, it will do two other things for you. First, it will give you your best chance of survival. When you feel good about others, feel good about yourself, and have a heart full of love, your immune system is going to go to bat for you. It will do everything it can to help that body of yours survive.

Second, even if it doesn't help you survive, it will give you the gift of a lifetime. It will give you a life that is much richer and more satisfying.

Whether I die before you read this or in another thirty years, I have achieved my purpose in life. I love, and I am loved.

CHALLENGE EXERCISES:

1. List five examples of times when people have shown you special caring since you have been diagnosed.

2. Above your list, write, "Five ways that I know that people care about me."

3. Take in the message of love that each of these acts of kindness represents.

4. Let these people know that you're grateful. You'll benefit as much from telling them as they will from hearing it.

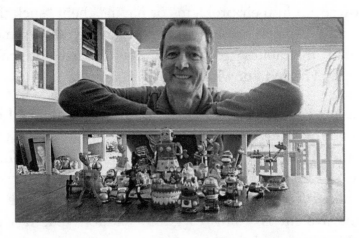

I loved it when my cousin Kevin brought me a wind-up robot. From there, the idea grew. This is what family and friends gave me for my 57th birthday.

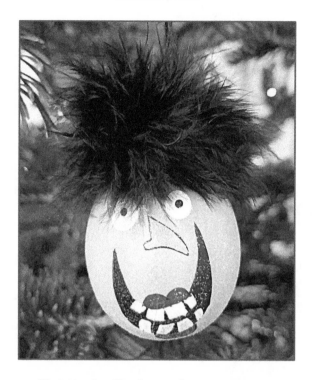

Christine's gift of a goofy egg ornament
brightens every Christmas.

CANCER IS A TEAM SPORT

Whatever affects one directly, affects all indirectly.

~ Martin Luther King, Jr.

Shortly after I was diagnosed with lung cancer for the first time, in 2006, Genevieve's cousin Barb and her husband, Dwayne, came to visit us in Portland. Dwayne had Stage IV cancer of the throat and had been dealing with cancer long enough to share his wisdom with me.

"The first thing you should know," he said, "is that when one person in the family has cancer, everyone in the family has cancer."

Dwayne was a very thoughtful guy, and he was clearly in his right mind, but I was a bit baffled by this comment. Cancer isn't contagious, so what did he mean?

He explained that the *impact* of cancer is felt by everyone in the family. How can it not be? Do you think your partner will just move along as if you are having your tonsils removed and not spend any more time worrying about it? Do you think that your children are avoiding you because what you are going through is unimportant, or because it is so important that they don't know what to do?

Go through the more distant branches on the family tree,

163

and you will still find those family members have the same concerns. We are part of something important, and all of the important people around us are impacted. Because of this, the whole family needs to be involved in some way.

Kevin, a friend from work, became very distressed when his father, Larry, developed esophageal cancer. Larry seemed depressed and uninterested in his upcoming treatment. Kevin immediately arranged a meeting between himself, me, and his parents to talk about attitude toward treatment.

We met at Kevin's favorite restaurant for coffee during off-peak hours, so we had a quiet spot where we were left alone. I was the last to arrive. Before I started talking, Larry already had his elbows on his knees, and his face was contorted with stress. He could barely say hello.

I started telling Larry about how attitude had made a difference in how effectively I have been able to deal with treatment, and how much it helped my mood. I gave him examples. The more I talked, the more he looked at the floor. He said nothing. Still, I continued. I knew I only had one shot to make sure he heard this.

I told him how much of a stress cancer had been on my family, and how I felt a responsibility to not only try to beat this cancer, but to have the best attitude possible, for their sake as well as mine.

By this time Larry's head was almost between his knees. I did what I could to revive his spirits. I gave him examples of times when I could see my family's, and particularly Genevieve's, spirits lighten because of my hopeful attitude under trying circumstances.

We ended our meeting. Kevin stayed to console his father, while I walked out with his mother, Beth. She thanked me for talking with Larry, but I apologized. Judging by the intense emotional reaction that I had just seen from Larry, I was afraid I had made things much worse. I felt depressed by having overwhelmed him with my words.

I was wrong about how Larry would respond. He really got the piece about how his attitude was impacting his entire family, specifically Beth, Kevin, and his grandchildren. It also helped when he understood that there was another way to approach his treatment and this phase of his life.

Larry did a complete turnaround and *thrived* during chemo. His attitude was outstanding. It probably won't come as a total shock to learn that his chemo was extraordinarily effective in shrinking his cancer. The last time I checked in, Larry had semi-retired, bought himself a '57 Chevy, and was cycling around the island of Kona.

Let's be clear about what happened. Larry's change in attitude wasn't because of any clever words on my part. In large part because Kevin and Beth had arranged what had amounted to a loving "intervention," and despite my blunt and fairly artless approach, Larry got the big picture: What he did from this point on made a tremendous difference to the people he loved.

There is no way of knowing how long Larry will live, but for the rest of their lives Larry's family will remember this part of Larry's life as a time to be celebrated. Larry was helped by his family, and Larry's family is forever changed by him.

So how will you impact your team?

The choice, my friend, is yours.

CHALLENGE EXERCISES:

1. Write down how you think your cancer has impacted each person in your family.

2. Have a discussion with them. This can be individually, or as a group. If they don't mention the items you have on your list, ask about them.

3. Write down what you have learned.

4. Reflect on whether there is anything that you now want to do differently.

OPENING THE DOOR (AND LEAVING IT OPEN)

Letting people in is largely a matter of
not expending the energy to keep them out.

~ Hugh Prather

In our everyday lives, many of us are insulated from needing to ask much of anyone we don't know well. We know pretty much just where we are going and what we are doing. We have clocks and GPSs in our phones, so we don't even need to ask for the time of day or for directions. But, by being so self-sufficient, we miss the opportunity to find out how kind and caring people really are.

Cancer changes all of that.

When we are diagnosed with cancer, it means that we are instantly and almost completely vulnerable. We lose our sense of control over our mortality, our bodily functions, our appearance, our ability to plan for the future. At times, we lack even the strength and energy to communicate.

We are not in charge. We weren't in charge before (despite what we thought), but now we're in charge even less.

In other words, we are blessed with needing other people to help us.

The goodness of human nature that has been buried in some of the people you know is going to surprise you. People that you thought were too tough-skinned or disconnected from the world to care will offer to do things for you, or say a kind word, while you watch the emotions you never knew they possessed sweep across their face.

There have been people that I didn't think would "get it" who have told me how moved they have been by something that I wrote. Occasionally, I have let one of my real estate clients know what I was going through. One of them, whom I didn't know very well at all, offered to do my grocery shopping for me or drive me to doctor's appointments. Other friends have cooked for us, given playful, silly, little gifts, prayed, visited, sent messages of support, and done anything else they could think of to tell me that they care.

It's not that I'm so extraordinary that people will go out of their way to help me. It's that many people are so extraordinary that they will find ways that most of us could never dream of to show that they care. All we have to do is to give them the opportunity to show us. Cancer is one of those opportunities. If you have cancer, don't let the opportunity pass you by.

Cancer breaks down the barriers for a lot of people. Just as strangers on the street will pat the belly of a pregnant woman (whether this is welcome or not), people who barely know me will go out of their way to do things for me when they know that I have cancer. All I have to do is to let them know what is going on, and to not rebuff their kindness.

I have found that when I share my life with others, they

find ways to share their lives with me. Different emails that I have sent out to family and friends have struck different people at different times. Sometimes, after I've sent out an email, a person that I haven't heard from in a year will respond, tell me that they have been thinking about me every day, and share a story about something moving that has happened: Sometimes it's about cancer or other health issues, and other times it's completely unrelated.

My friendships are deeper and stronger because I have been willing to share, regardless of whether my friends reciprocate. Every now and then, they do, and it's very special to me.

You can dare to ask for people to respond in a way you find helpful, whether it is a direct or indirect response you need. I did this at first by asking people to "think dried prunes" for me. I visualized the tumors shrinking up and looking like dried prunes. People did that for me, and told me about it. My friend Todd even gave me a bag of prunes with the message "I'm all in" written on the package. I also told people that the best kind of support for me was to avoid sympathy completely and to offer encouragement. People responded to that as well.

I tell you this as if it was an easy thing for me to do, and as if I can jump in and ask for what I need or want at any time. Not true. This is one of those lessons that I have to keep learning. For example, when I started radiation treatment in 2013, Genevieve went with me to the initial consultation, but she was going to be away at a five-day workshop with her twin sister on my first day in the clinic. That appointment is called a "simulation," and I would get scanned, probed, tattooed with reference marks for where the radiation would be aimed, and fitted with a form to hold my legs in the same position each time I was zapped. I was anxious about this but downplayed it because I didn't want Genevieve to miss her workshop.

That's when Lorin, my brother-in-law and closest friend, stepped in. He called and asked if I would like company. Going on autopilot, I told him, "No thanks," and treated it like it was no big deal. I had myself halfway convinced.

Lorin did the telephone equivalent of grabbing me by the lapels. "Listen," he said. "I'm offering you help and I want to be there. This is a bigger deal than you're letting on. You don't need to do this by yourself."

The wake-up call worked. I realized that this was a very emotional, vulnerability-inducing experience that I would either get through and remember in a very lonely way, or in a way in which I felt safe, supported, and even closer to a very close friend. A scary situation turned into one that enriched my life. Lorin, if you are reading this, thank you for this much-needed and timely reminder.

As you can see, learning to ask for and accept help has not been easy. I have often felt awkward, but I'm getting through it. I just have to keep reminding myself that *any* change is awkward. It doesn't mean it's a bad thing. It's just means that I'm not used to it yet. I'm also learning over and over again that getting used to changes isn't such a bad thing. Sharing what you are going through and asking for help ends up being helpful not only to you, but also to the people that you ask for help.

Here's an easy example: Have you ever had a five-year-old draw a picture and give it to you? This child feels like a million bucks for giving you this gift, because of the obvious pleasure it gives you. And the truth is, even if it isn't gallery quality, it feels pretty good when you look at it on your refrigerator.

Why is this so easy to recognize with kids and so hard to recognize with adults?

Rebbecca, a close friend, sends me an inspirational text message every evening before she goes to bed. She doesn't expect a response. She is sending healing thoughts my way, which she says is as good for her as it is for me. She says that it reminds her that the problems that she faces on a daily basis aren't really all that bad, and that there are other people in the world that have greater needs than she does. It helps her, she tells me, to feel grateful for the good life that she has.

I could say to her, "You're too kind. That's too much effort. You really shouldn't do that." But what would that do? I wouldn't be doing her any favors.

So, by accepting her gift, I'm also creating an opportunity for her to feel good. We are both giving, we are both receiving. We both feel closer, and we can both feel good that we have given each other something.

Keeping an open heart about accepting help from others is a gift to the giver AND to the one who receives.

CHALLENGE EXERCISES:

1. Make an email mailing list of everyone that you would want to give updates to about your health.

2. Send out an update on your health.

   a. Include whether the cancer is growing at this time, what treatment you are currently taking, and what comes next.

   b. Include the human side of your story: Share your fears and your hopes.

   c. Ask for what you need: Tell them how you want them to respond to you, such as support vs. pity, offering encouragement, including you in their prayers, visualizing dried prunes, etc.

   d. Specifically, ask for help if you need it.

3. If someone offers you help and your first reaction is to reject it, ask them if you can think about it for a bit. Next:

   a. List the reasons why you don't want to accept the help.

   b. List the ways you would benefit if you said yes.

   c. List the ways that the other person would benefit if you said yes.

   d. Weigh the choices. When in doubt, say yes.

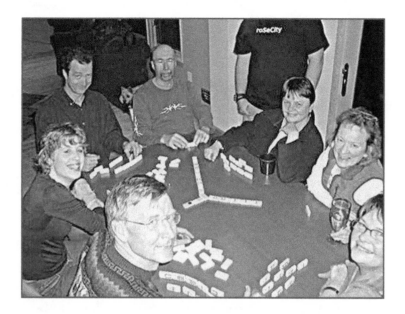

Clockwise from top: Jai Dev (up past his bedtime),
Ben (unfortunately headless), Genevieve, Rebbecca,
Charlotte, Lorin, Karen, me, and Kazul (on the cushion).

MAKING USE OF MY BEST FRIEND

To love yourself right now, just as you are,
is to give yourself heaven. Don't wait until you die.
If you wait, you die now. If you love, you live now.

~ Alan Cohen

One of the things that has made a very stressful situation much easier to cope with has been to have a best friend who is always looking out for my best interests. How can you not feel good about a person who makes sure that you have healthy food to eat? How can you not feel good about a person who finds opportunities for you to exercise, to stay in the best shape of your life in order to fight this beast? How can you not feel good about a person who compliments you on a job well done, reminds you to take it easy when you are pushing too hard, and forgives you for any mistake you make?

You may have guessed by now, but my new best friend has turned out to be me. I have been much kinder to myself since this cancer saga began. Whereas before I was a self-critical taskmaster who kept his nose to the grindstone, I am now much more of a cheerleader who is always looking for new ways to support myself.

I compliment myself for stepping out of my comfort zone to write a book, and to learn all the steps it takes to get it published. I forgive myself for not having the energy to work as hard as I used to, and for using bad judgment occasionally when merging in traffic, and for watching too much television. I pat myself on the back for being so consistent with my exercise, and for becoming more of an advocate for lung cancer survivors. I give myself a pass for occasionally having a mocha, or even for forgetting to take my cancer medication on a rare occasion.

Every time I give myself a pass, it feels great. Forgiveness is still so new to me that I feel like I am being extraordinarily kind just to not be self-critical. With every one of these caring kindnesses, it makes me feel better about being me.

Although I had been trying to move in this direction in therapy for years, I finally gave myself permission to go all-in being more nurturing when I needed it the most.

One of the outcomes of this has been that I am beginning to feel self-love. It's not because I've become really good at any particular thing. It's because I am being really good to myself.

As I mentioned in another chapter, if someone else treats me this well, I have struggled to believe it, or I would start wondering if I now owe that person something. Cancer has given me the opportunity to face these doubts. However, I don't have any of those issues when I am kind to myself. I trust the source.

Now is the time to treat yourself like an honored guest. While you still have the time.

CHALLENGE EXERCISES:

1. List three ways that you are supporting yourself in a kind way.

2. List the three most critical things that you say to yourself.

3. Think about the kind things that you would say to a good friend who was saying these critical things to himself/herself. This could be about forgiveness, or permission (telling the friend that he/she is allowed to make mistakes like everyone else), or acceptance of imperfection.

4. Write a letter to yourself that compliments you for each of the three ways that you are supporting yourself, and is kind to yourself in the three areas that you need it the most.

TALKING ABOUT DEATH

Friends share all things.

~ Pythagoras

Let's face it. Nobody wants to talk about death. That is, unfortunately, the problem. "Unpopular" is not a strong enough word. The topic itself, it seems, is as threatening as the Ebola virus.

Over the years I have heard people talk about their aging parents and grandparents. As soon as the elderly person brings up the unavoidable fact of death, a well-meaning child or grandchild will say, "Don't say that, Dad! You're going to live to be a hundred!" It doesn't matter if the elder is broaching the topic while in a hospital bed with monitors sounding alarms and IV lines hanging like marionette strings from poles. No, we don't say the "D" word out loud, because it will make it come true.

It's either that, or we can't talk about it because it makes us so uncomfortable.

I have been on both sides of this discussion. When I was thirty-four, my mother was diagnosed with pancreatic cancer, which was considered incurable at that time. After her diagnosis, we had several heart-to-heart discussions. In one of the earliest of these, I asked her to have professional photos taken while she still looked so good, so that I would always remember her in all her beauty. Those deeply personal discussions about her passions, her regrets, her family, and her hopes for my future will stay with me forever. And whenever I see those photos, I have loving memories of that time with her. One of these photos hangs directly outside of my bedroom door in the hallway, where I see it every time I walk out of my bedroom.

My stepfather, Vince, is in the final stages of Parkinson's disease. Discussions of dying with Vince have gone differently because we are both facing death, although his is more imminent. On my weekly visits, he often brings up the subject of his passing because he knows that I can truly comprehend what it is like. I see the sense of relief and the weight lifting from his shoulders as he shares his fears, his concerns for the future of his wife, Linda, and ultimately his acceptance of his circumstances. If I was to avoid these discussions, we would both be missing out on an opportunity to connect so deeply, and he would feel more isolated.

I understand the isolation part from firsthand experience. People want to talk with me about how I am going to live, but it is more challenging for them to explore with me what my death would mean. I feel isolated and alone in the world when this happens. The topic is too central to the very essence of having cancer to ignore.

Because the topic is so central, it is important to be able to tell your loved ones how crucial it is that they let you talk about it, if that is what you need. Even though Genevieve's belief in "creating your own reality" conflicts directly with talking about my death, she has at times been willing to take this step with me. I am grateful that she has been willing to accept that it is important to me, and that she remains open to me in what would otherwise become an increasingly lonely and isolating time.

Of course, sharing my thoughts and concerns with friends and family is easier when I am writing to them. It allows them to listen without interrupting long enough to understand, and sometimes to respond when something particularly poignant hits them. Usually this has occurred when I discussed my fear of death as some new symptom surfaced. Just having these fears acknowledged brightens my mood and lightens my load.

I hope you are able to find a way to talk with the people who are important to you about one of the biggest remaining taboo subjects. It's good for the soul. Whose soul?

The souls of both of you, of course.

CHALLENGE EXERCISES:

1. Think about who in your life you would most like the opportunity to talk with about death.

2. Rather than jumping directly into the discussion, ask the person if they are willing to let you share your thoughts about your possible death with them. Be prepared to reassure this person that talking about death won't make it happen. Help this person understand that not talking about it will leave you isolated in dealing with something that is very important to you, and that, if they

are willing to talk with you, the discussion will bring you closer.

3. If you have their permission, have the discussion.

4. At the end, ask permission to talk about it from time to time. This is not a one-time discussion.

VINCE

All you need is love.

~ John Lennon

My stepfather, Vince, has had Parkinson's disease for the past seventeen years. Over time, it has taken away almost all of his strength and muscle tone, to the point that he needs help getting into a wheelchair. His speech is barely audible in a quiet room if his dog's toenails are clacking on the linoleum. Even those of us who are closest to him have a hard time understanding his words anymore.

Parkinson's has also caused dementia. Formerly very articulate and a deep thinker, he now says very little during my visits because he gets lost in the middle of a sentence.

Vince and his wife, Linda, have been going to the same church for the past twenty years, but Vince has been unable to go for the past six months because the required physical effort is too draining. Last week, he rallied so that he could attend Easter services.

When I saw him later in the day, he was excited to tell me what had happened. In a blur of barely audible words and sentence fragments, he told me that dozens of people he knew had made a point of coming up to him after the service to say

183

hello, and to tell him how much they cared about him. As he told me this, his eyes puddled up and tears ran down his cheeks.

What had they said that was so magical that, even at a point when Vince can barely track the world around him, he was moved to tears? They told him the most important thing. By their presence, they told him that they love him.

Everything else is fading from his mind, but the power of love in his life remains.

This feels right to me. When I have gone through my darkest times dealing with cancer, it wasn't searching out survival statistics that kept me going. It wasn't reading books, watching television, doing exercise, having a healthy diet, or attending to my spiritual beliefs. It was knowing that I am loved.

I send my family and friends email updates on my health. Each time, many people that are close to me respond. They all give encouragement in one way or another. Sometimes they just call, or email, or drop by without any reason; but they let me know that they care.

Isn't that just another way of saying, "I love you"?

I believe that this message of love, in all its forms, is what has kept me alive.

CHALLENGE EXERCISES:

1. List as many ways as you can think of that people have

shown you love.

2. Add to this list regularly, as new ways come to mind.

3. If you know someone who might benefit from knowing that they are loved, say or do something to show it.

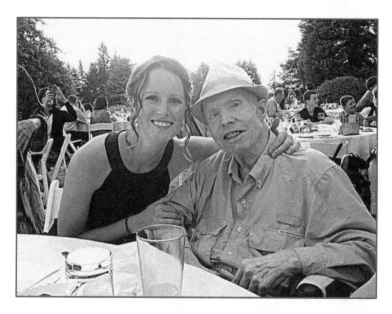

Vince with Stephanie, 2013

WALT

The mystery of human existence lies not in just staying alive,
but in finding something to live for.

~ Dostoyevsky

I have spent a lot of time over the eight years that I've had cancer thinking about the fact that some people are able to stay alive for much longer than anyone would expect. The example that shines brighter than all others for me is Walt, Genevieve's father.

Walt retired at the age of fifty-two, when the company where he worked was bought out. He puttered around with consulting, but had lost his direction and was floundering. That changed when he ended up raising Genevieve's son, Aidan. Walt volunteered for the job so Genevieve could have the opportunity to complete her college education. That decision changed three lives for the better.

Walt gave up consulting and focused his attention on Aidan. That included tutoring other children at Aidan's school, since Walt saw the need and no one else was filling it. He helped Aidan through college, and then through medical school. By taking on this "mission," he had helped out both Genevieve and Aidan, while taking a stand on one of his many values: "Get the best education that you can."

About the time that his mission with Aidan was finished, the health of his wife, Lorraine, started deteriorating. Walt gradually became her caregiver, and continued in this role right through her passing from ovarian cancer when he was eighty-four.

He was still playing tennis until about that time, but, as his body parts stopped cooperating, he scaled back to just the daily morning walks that he had been taking for decades.

Each day on those morning walks, he would see newspapers out near the sidewalk in front of the houses he passed. He would pick them up one by one, and hand-deliver them to the doorsteps of his neighbors. He never mentioned it to any of them unless they happened to see him, but he was looking after them nonetheless.

Walt stayed in touch with his college and army buddies through letters and occasional phone calls throughout his life — or at least throughout their lives: He outlived them all. One of these lifelong friends struggled financially, so, for decades, Walt sent this friend a little money on a regular basis.

When Walt's brother, Russell, and Russell's wife, Eloise, both died, Eloise's sister, Helen, had no family left. Her health and memory started declining, so Walt stepped in to manage her affairs for her. He and Lorraine would make the drive up from San Diego to Ventura to visit her and check in on her care a few times a year. They would stay overnight, then drive home the next day. He coordinated her transition into increasingly higher levels of care, until she passed away twelve years later.

During his retirement, Genevieve's twin sister, Charlotte, developed breast cancer. Walt saw it as his mission to help her get through this. He called her every day until she was out of the woods.

He also saw it as his mission to help his granddaughter Michele get through her pregnancies and the birth of her two children, though I'm still not quite sure what he considered his duties to be; most likely he was reminding her to get plenty of sleep and to eat well, but he took the job very seriously.

Not long after Lorraine passed away, Walt began volunteering for hospice. He was eighty-five at the time. Not surprisingly, a number of his "assignments" were younger than he was. He continued volunteering until he experienced a head trauma at the age of ninety-two.

After the head trauma, Walt was no longer able to live as independently, so, gradually, he accepted more in-home care. At this point, he announced that he had a new mission. That was to get up and do the best that he could to take care of himself, and to continue with his daily routines. One of his caregivers told me she loved working with him because he was one of the few people who would actually do all the recommended physical therapy exercises.

Walt also found another way to retain his dignity and sense of purpose. He considered his caregivers to be his staff. He was their employer and he was providing them with a good job.

So what was it that kept Walt alive until the age of

ninety-seven, even five years after a life-threatening head trauma?

Was it stubbornness? Walt could be stubborn, but I don't think that was it.

Was it just good genes? I think those helped, but in my mind there were even more important factors.

I think Walt's life was as long and rich as it was because he understood that it is important to have a purpose in life. I'm not sure that he would have articulated it this way, but in my mind his purpose was to take care of himself and the people he cared about in the best way he knew how.

Sometimes that was a kick in the pants, and sometimes that was a check in the mail. "You do what needs to be done."

This applied to neighbors as well as family, and even to shirttail relatives. "You take care of your people."

He had many missions in life, but they all seemed to come naturally to him. If you understand your purpose, knowing what your next mission should be will fall into place. You don't need to make it more complicated than it is.

Thank you, Walt, for your example of what a great life can look like.

CHALLENGE EXERCISES:

1. Reflect on your mission(s) in life.

2. Write down what you want your mission in life to be

from this point forward, whether you live for six months or thirty years.

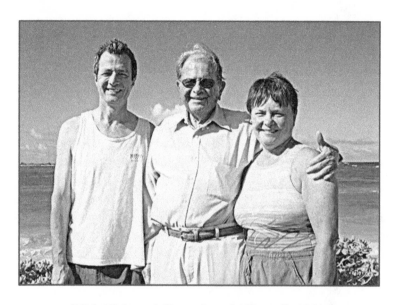

With Walt and Genevieve in Hawaii, 2010.
Walt was 92 in this photo.

A CAREGIVER'S PERSPECTIVE

It is not the load that breaks you down.
It's the way you carry it.

~ Lena Horne

Genevieve is an extraordinary person in so many ways. One of those is how she has handled being a caregiver. First, her identical-twin sister, Charlotte, got breast cancer. The connection between twins is much deeper than anyone who has not been around twins can imagine; the impact of one twin getting cancer is almost the same as if the other twin has gotten it, too. Not surprisingly, Genevieve spent a great deal of time with Charlotte during that very challenging stage of her life.

Nine years after Charlotte recovered, I developed lung cancer. Genevieve was by my side every step of the way as I survived those long odds and got through that battle. Then, just as it seemed I was out of the woods, Charlotte got breast cancer a second time. Of course, Genevieve went to every doctor's appointment and chemo session with her this time as well. A couple of years after that, my lung cancer returned. Once again, Genevieve was there for me through every step.

Nearly two years after I was diagnosed for the second time, her ninety-six-year-old father in San Diego started having mini-strokes and seemed to be nearing the end of his life. She called him daily and made trips to see him multiple times a year. Meanwhile, my stepfather, who lived ten minutes away, was in the final stages of Parkinson's disease and was not going to live much longer. I saw him every week, and Genevieve saw him fairly regularly.

If anyone was qualified to speak from the caregiver's perspective, it would be Genevieve. I asked her what she considered most valuable out of everything she had learned through her experiences.

What she told me made me laugh.

I laughed not because it was silly. I laughed because I had just spent the afternoon writing about how I had to learn the very same lesson.

The lesson is about letting go of control.

Genevieve has done everything within her power to make my cancer go away. She has been to every doctor's appointment and chemo session with me, and taken care of me when I needed it. She has tried to get me to supplement my medical care by connecting me with every kind of alternative health-care professional you can imagine, and then a few more. She put a crystal grid around our house. She created artwork designed to hit my optic nerve and send healing messages directly to my brain. She has tried hard to convince me that I can "will" the cancer away, if I just believe strongly enough.

In short, she has tried everything within her control to

make this cancer go away, and then she tried everything that is outside of her control.

In the end, she told me that she needs to keep reminding herself that, despite her efforts, she has no control over what happens to me. She can support me and encourage me, but, as she says (in her continuing effort to influence me), "It's your decision how long you stay on this planet, not mine."

She told me how hard it is to let go of the idea that she has control, because she wants so badly for me to stick around. She told me that all she can do is be a witness to my process rather than to be the force of change herself. She told me how hard it is to keep that in mind, because it's not how she wants things to be.

There are so many more issues as well, some of which she has told me about and some of which she has never said. She hates the thought of what it would be like to lose me, and also what it would be like to be alone again. She lives with constant uncertainty about my future, our future, and her future. She has worried about how she will manage some of the tasks in our life that I take care of, like changing furnace filters and turning off the water to the outside faucets so that the pipes don't freeze in the winter. She would have to manage her finances without my help, and suffer the loss of my income.

Because I am the one with cancer, all the support comes to me, yet her life is being turned upside down as well. How can she get the support she needs? Under any other circumstances, the first place she would go for support would be to me. However, she worries that she will be putting more

195

of a load on me, or that her doubts will rub off on me, or that I will spend too much time worrying about how she is doing. I am extremely grateful that she has Charlotte to talk with, and even more so (for this reason only) that Charlotte has dealt with cancer twice herself.

When people realize how much Genevieve is also going through, some of them ask her how she is doing. She finds the question very difficult to answer, because, as I have experienced myself, she doesn't know if they are just saying hello in a generic social way, really want to know, or are somewhere in between. It's a much tougher question than you would think. (I've written about it as a separate topic elsewhere in this book, in the chapter titled, "How Are You?")

Genevieve shared another very important piece. She told me that, while being a caregiver so many times, the most valuable coping skill that she has learned has been to "stay on the page of today." There are enough problems for any of us to deal with in the present, without piling on problems that may not ever happen.

CHALLENGE EXERCISES FOR THE CAREGIVER:

1. List all of the ways that you try to help your partner live longer.

2. Next to each, mark whether you have *control* or *influence* over whether they get done.

3. Tell your partner what it feels like to be in the caregiver role.

4. Put an asterisk next to any items that have created

tension between you and your partner. What causes the tension? List all that apply:

a. Your partner dislikes being told what to do.

b. There is a difference in how important or relevant each of you considers the item.

c. You are trying to *control* something that can only be *influenced*, and even then, only with the cooperation of your partner.

5. Discuss the list with your partner.

a. Remind your partner that you do these things both because you love them and want them to live, and because you don't want to be left alone.

b. Tell your partner that you understand that these are their decisions to make, not yours, even though it is very hard for you to not have control.

6. Discuss the differences you may have in how important or relevant each of you considers some of the items.

7. See the table "National Resources for Lung Cancer" at the end of this book. On a blog site that feels comfortable for you, search out or start a discussion on what it is like to be a caregiver.

8. Ask your local cancer center if they have resources for caregivers.

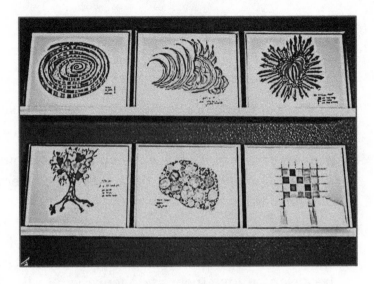

Just a fraction of the artwork that Genevieve
has created to set me on a healing path

LOVE AND THE BOUNDARIES
OF ACCEPTING HELP

We love life, not because we are used to living
but because we are used to loving.

~ Friedrich Nietzsche

We all have our own theories about what may help us survive cancer. Of course, there are the medical treatments, and if they were 100 percent successful, that would be the end of the story. For example, if a person's heart stops, using defibrillators is the treatment of choice. You don't hear people recommending homeopathic cures or praying for the heart to start again on its own. But with cancer, the cure is not so certain, so we look for any way we can control what prescribed treatment cannot.

My cancer has forced many people that I care about to cope with a great deal of discomfort. They can't stand not being able to fix this thing for me. I get it. It feels helpless to be out of control. So they do what well-meaning people everywhere do: they offer everything that they can think of. Loved ones have given me diets to try, tapes to listen to, stacks of books and articles to read, encouragement to join their religion, websites for yoga that heals – whatever they can think of that might help. They have suggested acupuncture, remote healing, and clinics in Mexico. They have prayed for me in synagogues, churches, and homes. Those who don't pray have sent positive thoughts my way. Crystal grids have been set around our house, and even aliens have been called upon.

Then there are the more direct approaches: People have made phone calls, sent emails, and dropped by with soup. They have spent time with me and told me that they cared in so many ways. Here is what I think about this:

It's all love, and it's all working. Love is keeping me alive.

A casual acquaintance took the time to research an article on a cancer-stopping diet for me. I didn't think the diet would work, but how could I not be touched by this man's attempts to help me? My stepmother, Linda, had "Livestrong" style wristbands with my name made up and gave them to family and friends to wear. How could my heart not swell with the love I was being shown? Why should it matter if these people have the same spiritual beliefs as me? It's all love. It's all love.

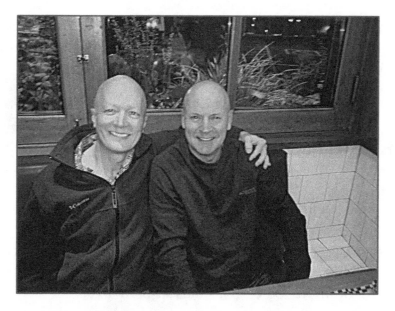

My friend Buck showing love in a big way: He shaved
his head bald in support while I went through chemo.

But can love really keep you alive?

I remember reading in a college psychology class about
an orphanage in Germany during World War II. Due to severe
staffing shortages, the babies were fed but not held. Many of
them died due to what was called "failure to thrive
syndrome." Also from my vault of college memories, baby
monkeys raised in isolation were given the choice of either a
warm fuzzy monkey doll or a steel monkey-shaped cage that
contained food. They chose to starve rather than give up the
comfort of the warm contact. What does this tell us? We
would rather die than be without love.

I am convinced of this. I am certain that if I had been
diagnosed with cancer when I was still in my previous,

unhappy marriage, I would have been dead long ago. It would not have been worth going through everything you need to go through to beat cancer.

Now it is just the opposite. Against long odds, I'm still here eight years after first being diagnosed. Without Genevieve to love and support me, I wouldn't have found the inner strength to strive for life.

Genevieve is a part of this, but it has taken all of the parts together to keep me alive. Feeling the prayers and positive thoughts, the expressions of caring and the acts of kindness from everyone around me nurtures my soul every day. All of this together gives me reason to live.

My friend Chaz told me that, shortly before his father died, his father said that he had received the greatest gift of his lifetime. His children taught him that he was lovable. I think he was on to something.

However, the issue is more complicated than just accepting every kind of help offered. Often these well-meaning people want me to change my own behavior in ways that they believe might help.

I have gone through enough chemo, radiation, and surgery to tell you that, in order to recover, every one of these treatments requires an enormous amount of energy and time. I am sure that the same is true for immunotherapy and other forms of treatment. While these are all gifts of love, and I appreciate them, there are many paths to take, and all of them are different than the path that I am already on.

At first I found it hard not to feel guilty that I didn't read every article and book given to me. I didn't have it in me to research whether radon had affected my lungs or whether remote healing was going to make the cancer disappear. Every new option would require that I make some important change. But these suggestions always seem to be offered at the critical points in treatment when my health has just gone through another major change, when I have been under the most stress, and when most of my limited remaining energy is going toward recovering from treatment. There were times that I barely had the energy to get out of bed.

I came to the conclusion that I couldn't try to change just to placate other people, even people very close to me. I decided instead that my best path to success would be to trust myself. Did it feel right when someone suggested I give up all dairy products? Was an herbal supplement going to change my life? If my instincts said no, I said no.

Sometimes my gut says yes, so I say yes. It was reasonable for Genevieve to suggest that I take turmeric every day, since there is a consensus forming that it may have anti-cancer properties. I switched my oral diabetes medication to metformin, since at least some research supports using it to fight lung cancer. I also started taking a therapeutic dose of melatonin every night, since I had discovered that there were clinical trials underway to determine the effectiveness of melatonin in fighting lung cancer. These are the kinds of things that I ask my doctor about before starting, however, since I don't want to do anything that interferes with treatment that is proven to be effective.

I am more willing to try things that I have doubts about

if someone important to me is asking, and especially if the ratio of effort-to-reward is agreeable. For example, Genevieve wanted me to use a "healing mat." This mat is big enough to lie down on and is filled with amethyst crystals. Infrared light projects through the crystals, generating light waves that are purported to have a healing frequency. I'm not sure at all about the healing frequency, but it also generates warmth. Almost every evening I lie down on this ~~heating pad~~ "healing mat." Genevieve feels better that I am using it, and so do I.

When I don't agree with the suggestions, it has taken some practice for me to accept whatever the latest advice is without committing to trying it. I express my appreciation for the advice-giver's intentions, try to keep an open mind, and show at least a little interest in the suggestion. If pressed, I might go as far as to nod and say, "I might look into it." At times, when pressed even further, I have learned to be more direct. I say that it may work for some people, but doesn't feel right for me. When really pushed, I have had to say, "I have a lot on my plate right now. There's only so much that I can take on. I have to do what feels right to me."

It seems to me that when people push too hard, it's because they forget that this is about my needs and not theirs. It doesn't matter how "right" someone else is. I'm the one who has to decide what is right for me.

I understand how people get into that encouraging, almost pushy mode. Someone close to me was telling me that she might not complete follow-up treatment after her cancer was surgically removed. The treatment didn't improve the survival odds much, and the side effects could be pretty severe and would last for a very long time. I tried to convince her that she should do everything she could to increase her survival odds. She shrugged off my encouragement and made her own decision. After I realized what I had done, I called her up and gave her support for making a decision that was right for her.

Sometimes people (myself included) just need to be reminded about whose agenda it is.

However...

Even though it's my own agenda, desperation has tempted me to try many things beyond my comfort zone. I learned that staying true to what I believe will work for me is one of the hardest skills to master, and one of the most important. But the disease and the treatment (and sometimes the emotional toll) drain my energy, and there are only so many paths I can take. So how do I stay on track?

Yes, it's important to keep an open mind, but you also have to believe in yourself. You have to put everything you have into taking the steps that *you* think will work. If you're not sure, or if you keep changing directions, your focus gets diluted. The more miracle cures you chase, the more desperate the search feels.

It's a whole lot easier to believe in yourself if you have someone else who believes in you as well. That person doesn't have to believe exactly as you do, just to respect that you will make the best decision for yourself after taking everything in. Genevieve has done that for me in an extraordinary fashion. She has very strong opinions about alternative paths to health. I take in what fits, and then I remind her that it has to be me that makes the choices. When Genevieve steps back and remembers this, she becomes the world's greatest cheerleader. She backs me up with everything she has. And here is something that she does that is extremely helpful when I'm struggling: She reminds me of what I do that is working, such as writing about what I am experiencing, and then encourages me to keep at it.

There is more than one path to health. Some paths feel right for me, and some feel absolutely wrong, though they may be perfect for someone else. If my heart isn't in it, my feet aren't going to follow for very long. My energy is too precious to do anything other than to follow my own path.

CHALLENGE EXERCISES:

1. List all the things that people have offered as help that do not require you to do anything.

2. Write down everything that you appreciate about these actions.

3. Tell these friends and loved ones what you appreciate.

4. Think of an <u>unwanted</u> suggestion someone has made that would require you to take some action.

5. Write down what you appreciate about the intentions of the person offering the help, even if you didn't appreciate the pressure to do what this friend or loved one is urging you to do.

6. Write down how you would tell the "helper" that you are not going to try what they have recommended. Here's an example: "Thank you for suggesting that I

_____. I really appreciate your thinking about me. However, that one doesn't feel like a good fit for me. My plate is pretty full right now, and I only have enough energy to do the things that are at the top of my priority list."

7. Ask a friend or loved one to role-play with you.

8. Practice in real life as needed.

GENEVIEVE

Love must be as much a light, as it is a flame.

~ Henry David Thoreau

I have written a lot about the importance of love in all its forms, about its being crucial to my continuing to succeed at cancer. I believe it may even be keeping me alive. My relationship with my wife, Genevieve, who is mentioned often throughout this book, has been the purest, richest form of this love in my life.

The outpouring of her love, and the sharing of my love with her, heals me in a way that nothing else could. Genevieve is my wish come true for this lifetime.

Love is not the only reason that I am still succeeding, and possibly living longer, after almost nine years with cancer, but it is the most important. It is also what makes life worth living.

Understanding that love is keeping me alive does not put weight on the relationship. Neither of us believes that Genevieve is responsible for what happens to me. We have this discussion often, because it is so important for both of us to keep this in mind. Also, her importance doesn't leave me feeling needy; it just gives me more reason to feel grateful.

I don't believe that it is necessary to have such a rich and meaningful relationship to succeed at cancer. It helps tremendously, however.

Whether or not you have such an extraordinary relationship, it certainly helps to have all kinds of rich and meaningful relationships. It is especially helpful if you can have a relationship like this with yourself, whether it starts out that way or not.

I hope that you are blessed with such relationships. Whether you are already blessed in this way or not, I also hope that you can create more along your journey.

CHALLENGE EXERCISES:

1. If you are blessed with such a loving relationship, let the person you love know how much they mean to you, and how much you appreciate them.

2. Repeat #1 frequently. It takes little energy, and you will get back more than you give. Every time.

3. If you are in a relationship, but it is more strained than this:

   a. Let go of what you can. Your life is too important, and your time is too precious, to let things get in the way.

   b. Consider couples counseling.

   c. On one sheet of paper, write down all of the things that you appreciate about your partner. On another, list all of the things that bother you.

d. On the "bother" list, try a fresh perspective. Which of these items are minor in the big picture? Which of these have been more pronounced since you were diagnosed, and can be chalked up to the considerable stress? Which of these can you talk about?

e. Burn the "bother" list and focus on the "appreciation" list.

PART III:

TAKING ACTION

REMOVING THE CANCERS

I will not let anyone walk through my mind with their dirty feet.

~Mahatma Gandhi

Cancer has definitely led to a reevaluation of my priorities. I have made a lot of changes since I was diagnosed, but one of the most important things that I decided to do was to eliminate the "cancers." I cannot afford to be around people who have a corrosive influence on my spirit.

I hadn't been doing anything all that self-destructive, but some of my choices just weren't healthy. It's like eating junk food. A little bit isn't a problem, is it? Well, maybe it is.

There were people that I spent time with who just didn't treat me with the kind of love and respect that I give to others. I decided that I deserved the same respect, and I wasn't going to put up with anything less. I stopped worrying so much about hurting someone else's feelings and started thinking about how unhealthy it was for me to be around critical people who undermine me. Hanging around with these people would be like hanging around someone with a bad cold during chemo, when my immune defenses were down. Why would I compromise myself like that?

Why do I need to give my time to people who don't

215

value me enough to treat me well? Why do I need to be with people who walk through life with a bitter taste in their mouths? What do I get from being with people who expect the worst from others, and have a knack for rooting it out?

Occasionally, you may run into people like this, but your lives are so intertwined that completely eliminating them from your life may create more problems than it solves. At least for me, I found that if I went into those situations with a different attitude, I could still come out unscathed. Just like the battleships from Star Trek, I come in with my shields up. I keep the conversation superficial, avoid controversial topics, and expect nothing back. These people no longer disappoint, because I realize that that was all I was going to get back from them anyway. By changing my attitude and approach, I have isolated the cancer in my life, if not removed it completely. That works for me.

It gets harder when the people who fall into this category are family members, but that makes it even more important to find a way to deal with them. For example, at one point I sent out an email telling family and friends that the cancer had just spread further in my lungs, and had for the first time spread beyond my lungs and into my bones. I asked for support at this very vulnerable time. Instead, one family member responded with the most hurtful email possible. He chose this point of greatest vulnerability to attack me about things that had happened two decades earlier between us. I had to tell him that I loved him, but that I would have no further contact with him. I explained that I did not have the energy to defend myself when I barely had enough energy to stay alive.

There were others, including another family member

that was even more scathing, but who directed this venom at several people. That situation was easier to see coming, so I had already minimized contact and distanced myself. There is not an easy way to eliminate contact with this person without severing relationships with the rest of the family, so I show up and keep my invisible shields in place.

Television can also be another source of negativity. I still watch it, but I choose what I watch with a more careful eye. I won't watch shows that are saturated with terror and torture. I won't waste a minute of my time on "reality" shows in which disturbed people get attention for insulting, backstabbing, and manipulating each other. These are cancers around us. I am not going to feed them, and they are not going to feed on me.

A variation on this theme: The people who have come up to me and said that they are *so sorry* that I am going through this, and then spend the next half an hour telling me how hard my cancer has been for them to deal with because they feel *so bad* about it. It's not my job to hear how it makes them suffer, or to make them feel better about my cancer.

People like this can suck the life out of you by making everything – *everything* – about them. There is a technical name for these people. They are called "Energy Vampires." OK, so it's not a technical term. But it should be. You cannot afford to have your energy drained. This will not help you to survive.

There is no easy way to change the behavior of Energy Vampires, since this is how they live their entire lives. The best way to cope is to minimize contact with them, or avoid them altogether. A friend told me that a woman from her church came up to her when she found out about her diagnosis. This woman told my friend that she knew someone else who had gone through the same thing, "and I stayed with her right up to the end. Now I'm going to do the same for you." My friend told me that her first thought was, "oh, no, you're not!"

If you have cancer, your immune system is already compromised. You cannot be around people who bring with them the emotional equivalent of a cold. I have managed cancer quite well, but colds have kept me feeling bad for up to three months at a time on several occasions. Don't let the Energy Vampires give your life a cold. You need everything you have in order to deal with cancer.

There are other "cancers" out there as well. People usually consider cancer blogs to be inspirational, although I have found that sometimes this is not the case. There are people who want to tell you just how hard their life is, but they don't offer anything helpful or hopeful. Some of these blogs elicit nothing but pity. How is that going to inspire anyone? I encourage you to be selective about what sort of influence from bloggers you want to absorb before you go down the rabbit hole.

The daily news can be another cancer in our lives. The focus is on car, plane, and train crashes, fires, rapes, murders, wars, and political bickering.

Someone once said that if you get away from the media and college campuses, life isn't so depressing after all. I find that pre-recording the news and then fast-forwarding through the parts I view as cancerous makes the news much more valuable to me.

And shorter. Much, much, shorter.

CHALLENGE EXERCISES:

1. Make a list of the cancers in your own life.
2. Next to each, write down how you want to deal with that cancer going forward.
3. You know what comes next.

EXERCISE: THE WONDER DRUG

Exercise should be regarded as tribute to the heart.

~ Gene Tunney

One of the best things that I have done for myself throughout these eight years has been to exercise. I climb the seven flights of stairs up to my office twice a day. I go to the gym five days a week. I take walks after work when there is enough daylight and the rain isn't too heavy. For cardio activity, I shoot baskets and run around chasing missed three-pointers. If you knew how many shots I missed, you would be impressed with just how aerobic this activity is.

Both times before I had lung surgery, I stepped it up. I considered myself to be in training for surgery, so I upped my cardiac workouts and did more core strength exercises. My back gets sore easily, so I thought I would have an easier time lying in the hospital bed for days if I strengthened my back and all the supporting muscles. Once out of the hospital, I started with walking and progressed to the gym at the first opportunity.

There are so many benefits to exercise that if it came in pill form, it would be a bigger hit than Viagra. Well, close, anyway. First, it does wonders for the mood. I notice it when I exercise, but I notice it a whole lot more when I don't. I don't have as much energy, my mood is a little flat, and my attitude takes more work. I have more energy to *want* to do things when I have been exercising regularly.

It is excellent for building stamina. Now that my lungs are compromised, it takes a lot more energy to do any kind of activity. When I've had some minor muscle tweak or something has kept me from exercising for two or three weeks, I notice how much more easily I get winded. It comes back pretty quickly, though, once I get some activity going again. I noticed the stamina part a great deal when I was recovering from surgery and when I went through chemo. I accepted that I was going to be on the sofa for one and a half days during each chemo cycle, but for the rest of the days, my nursing staff was always surprised at how active I remained. The only thing I was doing differently from anyone else was that I was exercising.

I also *feel* stronger when I'm exercising, because I *am* stronger. All I have to do is take a vacation from exercising and then try to lift the same weights when I get back in the gym to see how much difference regular exercise makes.

Exercise also boosts the immune system. Every form of cancer treatment is some form of assault on the body, making it easier for you to get sick from something unrelated to cancer. The last thing I wanted when I was already taking my licks was to get double-teamed by some bug. Even though I was almost overly cautious about avoiding germs, I still got colds that lasted for three months. I wonder how much worse it would have been if I didn't have my immune system in the best possible shape to fight it.

The benefit of exercise that makes the most difference to me, however, is the one that is intangible. I may not be able to control the outcome of treatment, but I can definitely take charge of taking care of myself. When I do that, I can see tangible results and know that I am giving myself the best possible chance to survive.

Here's how it looks to me: Whatever treatment you try is hard on your body. Most of the time it doesn't kill all the cancer, so you need to either repeat that treatment or go through another treatment that is also hard on your body. That can only happen after you are in good enough shape to take on the next hit. The longer you take to recover, the more time the cancer has to grow.

In short, you have a better chance of fighting off cancer if you are in the best shape possible and can rebound quickly after each treatment. How do you get in the best shape possible, with the best stamina, strongest immune system, and the most energy? There are a few factors, but a big one is exercise.

Show me a drug that can match what exercise does: Makes you faster, stronger, healthier, quicker to recover; increases your stamina; helps you feel more in charge of your life; and improves your mood. Oh, and there's one other plus:

All of the side effects are positive.

CHALLENGE EXERCISES:

1. List exercise options that you enjoy, and realistic options for your own situation.

2. Consult with your doctor or other health-care provider to adapt these exercises to your abilities and your health condition.

3. Do your exercise routine for at least fifteen to twenty minutes each time.

4. Gradually build up the length and the frequency to as much as you can tolerate. Ideally, this will be daily.

5. Once you have done #3, and then again after #4, congratulate yourself for taking such good care of yourself.

SAY YES MORE OFTEN

Why do you stay in prison, when the door is so wide open?

~ Rumi

For many of us, when we're in our teens and twenties we think we're going to live for another hundred years. Risks don't seem that big a deal, because we think nothing is going to happen to us. It will happen to the other guy. Gradually or suddenly, we experience enough to change our mind and decide that life is a little more precious. It's still hard to accept that life is not as limitless as air, however.

There's still plenty of time to start a new career, patch up a damaged relationship, or take up a new hobby, right? Well, what happens if there is not? Will you have any regrets?

I've lived a lot of my life not knowing what I wanted, and yet I was too emotionally shut down to even guess at what it might be. Now, with a new sense of urgency, I'm learning that there may be ways of finding out.

I read "Yes Man," a book by Danny Wallace which was later made into a movie with Jim Carrey. The main character, who has become shut down and disconnected from his friends, hits rock bottom. His relationships are getting seriously harmed by his isolation. When he finally decides he needs to do something different, he goes to the extreme. He vows to say *yes* to everything that anyone asks of him. This decision has a major impact on his finances, his relationships, and his career.

It's all very funny when it happens in a book or in the movies, but that solution was a bit extreme for me. However, I liked the concept so much so that I made the only New Year's resolution that I can ever remember making:

Say YES more often.

I did it for a year. You know what? It works. I discovered that my natural reflex was to say *no*. "That won't work because..." "I wouldn't like that because..."

During that year, I tried many things that I didn't love. But I liked many more than I had thought I would. I went sailing with my friend Todd on his boat. I signed up for the half-court basketball shot to win a car at the Blazer game; I wasn't selected, but the anticipation made it more exciting, and I started practicing half-court shots at the gym, just in case. It added some more fun to my life.

I also learned to take risks. Not the bungee-jumping or skydiving variety. The risks were more of the "I'm-going-to-tell-people-what-I-really-think" variety. This is not the same as being critical of people in the name of honesty, which is actually pretty selfish. It's more along the lines of sharing my opinions and trusting that someone will care. For example, letting a group of friends know that I don't want to go to the theater that they all love, because I'm tired of simplistic boy-meets-girl, happily-ever-after plays. I'll compromise with them, but I won't hide my opinion. I will also tell them that I'd rather we all went for a bike ride rather than go downtown to watch the parade. When the situation arises, I will also occasionally share my liberal political views in an office full of conservatives. It's not earth-shattering, but for some of us, standing out from the crowd is very uncomfortable.

And you know what I found out? Most people like me better when I tell them what I think.

What a surprise.

At an art show, Genevieve and I found a quote by Anaïs Nin, which was carved into a clay tile. It now hangs from my wall:

"Life shrinks or expands in proportion to one's courage."

I love this quote. I look at it every time I'm writing emails to family and friends about my health. I use it as inspiration to share much more than just a medical report, to share what is important to me. When I have doubts about sticking my neck out (all the time), I also get a much-needed gentle nudge from my therapist and from Genevieve. Every time, I have taken their advice and taken the risk. Every time, the feedback has been positive. Yet I still have a lifetime of self-doubt to overcome.

Take this book, for example. It feels like a massive risk to me to write a book about myself, and about my ideas. I have a hard enough time believing that anyone wants to hear what I say in a normal conversation unless I keep it very brief. I'm still surprised every time I write an email to family and friends and someone tells me that they love what I write. How can I believe strangers would want to read a whole book, when it's hard for me to believe that people who are already close to me want to read a two-page email?

What I have finally decided is that I have something to say that is important for me to share, regardless of whether anyone else agrees. Even if I write for an audience of one, it has been worth the effort.

What you say *yes* to will probably be different than what I say *yes* to. Regardless, I'm betting you'll end up with a richer life because you tried.

Say YES more often.

CHALLENGE EXERCISES:

1. List the last five things that people have invited you to do. This could be as simple as asking to come over to your house to visit you. If you can't think of five, keep adding to the list as new invitations come up.

2. Write down how you responded to each one.

3. Consider how things would be different if you had chosen the other option (no instead of yes, or yes instead of no).

4. Moving forward, consider saying yes more often.

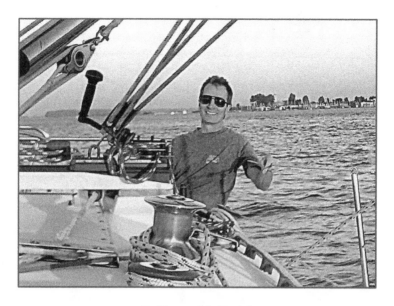

Sailing with Todd

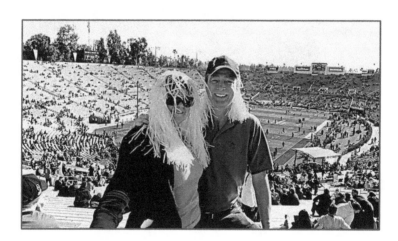

Soaking up the atmosphere at the Rose Bowl with Genevieve

MAKING BAD CHOICES (FEELS GOOD)

Everything in moderation, including moderation.

~ Oscar Wilde

I know all the healthy things to do for myself. They include diet, exercise, doctor visits, sleep, attitude, spirituality. It doesn't take much work to figure this out, and I'm highly motivated to do these things. Still, here's my little secret:

I don't always make the healthy choice, and I feel good about it.

I normally don't tell people this part, for obvious reasons. They might gasp and say, "Isn't sugar *bad* for cancer?" or "You didn't go to the gym today? I thought that was an important part of your fight against cancer." They would be right. There's more to it than that, and it's not easy to explain.

There is no doubt that making the healthy choice 100 percent of the time is better for my body. However, if I make that choice 100 percent of the time, it stops being a choice. It becomes an unbreakable rule, even a law. I would start to feel like I was in prison. I would no longer feel good about doing it. I would feel trapped and resentful.

There's enough on my plate already without feeling trapped by the responsibility of always making the perfect choice. That would be cancerous.

231

Instead, I live with something I learned after being diagnosed with diabetes about ten years ago. I learned to live by the 95 percent rule: It's what you do 95 percent of the time that really matters. (If you are a brittle diabetic, this is probably very bad advice. Take this with a grain of salt – not sugar.)

The related piece of this is that I feel much better about myself if I'm OK with whatever choice I make.

I really can have my cake and eat it too.

CHALLENGE EXERCISES:

1. Think of one thing that you *feel* you have to do, while you *know* that if you skipped it once, it wouldn't matter. (NOTE: Do not skip medical treatment. Try something less drastic.)

2. Skip it once.

3. Write down what it felt like, and whether you would ever want to have that as an option again. Be careful: This is not an invitation to become inconsistent – just enough to feel like you have a choice.

LIVING WITH A DEADLINE

You may delay, but time will not.

~ Benjamin Franklin

You certainly didn't want it, but you have been given an incredible gift. You have been reminded in the most in-your-face way possible that you are not immortal. This may not be what you asked for, but in many ways this is a good thing.

Have you ever had a test and waited until the last minute to study? How about a report that you had to turn in? Cleaning up the house just before company arrives? You get the idea.

Most of us do our most focused work under pressure of time. Some of this work we would never get around to unless there was a deadline. Not only are you not immortal, but it's possible you may not have much time left. Maybe it's time to finish your homework.

If you knew that you had one year to live, what would you do? The usual things that many people imagine are taking a trip around the world or buying expensive toys because "you can't take it with you."

I haven't come up with one clear answer, but I am getting closer. I'm taking care of the things that are important to me. I'm letting the people that I am closest to know how much they mean to me. I'm doing my best to get my affairs in order so that Genevieve will have an easier transition if I die. I'm clearing the garbage out of my life so that I can give my energy to what is most important to me. I'm trying to have more experiences that are meaningful, enriching, or memorable. As I've mentioned elsewhere, I'm removing the cancers from my life. I'm trying to get to know myself better. One of the ways I do this is by writing, which helps me to clarify my thinking.

The core of what I am focusing on is having closer relationships with people I am already close to. It turns out that the way to do this is not a big secret. I just tell them what I'm going through and how I feel about it, and I ask them about their lives.

I remain as open as I can be to the possibility of being close to more people. Why should I limit myself from being connected with anyone? Have I passed my expiration date for making new friends? What opportunities will I miss out on if I live for another thirty years? Wouldn't cutting myself off cost me something great, even if I die in six months?

The part that is harder for me to understand is that other people are willing to get closer to me. They understand the possibility that I may not be alive for very long. It's human nature to protect yourself against the pain of loss, and to withdraw or not get close to people who aren't going to stick around.

As an example, it often takes time for some people to be willing to make friends when you go to a new place, because they want to see if you're going to hang around before they extend themselves. Despite my cancer, I have been surprised at how little of this self-protection I have seen from people around me. Staying engaged is making my world a little better every day. I'm much happier than I have ever been in my life.

CHALLENGE EXERCISES:

1. Make a list of your most important values, and how these values show up in your life.

2. Make a "bucket list" that is in line with your values.

3. Start taking action steps, even if they are small steps, towards achieving those goals.

BEING YOUR OWN ADVOCATE

If opportunity doesn't knock, build a door.

~ Milton Berle

Most of what I have talked about so far has to do with attitude. Sometimes that's not enough. At times you will need to make active choices and take pure, no-holds-barred action.

There are many decision points that you may not even recognize over the course of living with cancer. Each of them can be critical in your survival, and making the wrong decision, or being passive, can cost you your life. My own mistakes almost cost me mine.

While some decisions that I made were sound, at times I got help. When I was first diagnosed, Genevieve and my friend Rebbecca, both of whom worked in a hospital, searched around and found the top lung cancer specialist in the Northwest for me. This doctor and I clicked immediately, in part because we both had the same "take no prisoners" approach to attacking the cancer.

Next, Genevieve, Rebbecca and I found two top lung surgeons in the area. Genevieve and I interviewed both of them and compared their different surgical approaches (open-chest versus minimally invasive), I read about the pros and cons of these approaches online, and then I chose a surgeon that I believe was excellent.

Partly because of those two choices, and partly because I chose to be treated with the most aggressive chemo cocktail possible, I became cancer-free for almost five years. So far, so good.

Halfway through this blissful period, I made my first potentially life-threatening decision, which in truth was a passive non-decision. My oncologist left the state, so the clinic assigned me to another oncologist. I accepted this doctor without asking questions or checking his credentials. Even after not liking his vague, non-committal answers over the course of many appointments, I stuck with him. HUGE mistake on my part. I admit it: I was passive because I wanted to believe that I was cancer-free, and therefore his qualifications were no big deal.

I couldn't have been more wrong.

After almost five years in remission, when I had my first CT scan that showed something unusual in my lungs, this oncologist was baffled. He said he didn't know what it was, but that it didn't look like cancer. His advice: Wait and see what happens with the next scan. AGAIN I was passive, and I agreed. This was my second big mistake, and this one could have gotten me killed.

If there was something growing in my lungs, why would there be any question whether it should be investigated immediately? The stakes were too high for a game of wait-and-see. Yet that's what he suggested, and that's what I went along with. Four months later, the new scan showed that the already-countless spots were growing larger, and that there were more of them. This time he suggested a biopsy. He thought it could be bacteria, or lupus, or tuberculosis – cancer was unlikely. "But if it is cancer," he said, "call the clinic and ask them to refer you to someone else, because I'm not a lung cancer specialist."

WHAT? Then what had he been doing treating me all this time? Never mind that he wouldn't even refer me himself – I was stunned by his eleventh hour admission. I was angry with him for treating me all this time, but even more upset with myself for not checking his credentials.

After finding out that I not only had lung cancer, but also that it was Stage IV, I called the clinic and left an urgent message that I needed to get in to see a lung cancer specialist. Several days later, I got a message back: "Hi, I understand that you want to make an appointment. Please call again." Here I was, again passive, thinking that the thoughtful doctors behind the scene had been contemplating who would be the best fit. Instead, it had taken that long for the support-staff person to get around to returning my phone call. I left another message, again expressing my urgency.

By the next day, Genevieve had seen where this was going, and took charge. She consulted with a friend in the medical community, who gave her the names of two oncologists – at a different clinic – that her friend thought were the top two options in the city at that time. I stopped waiting for the non-responsive clinic, and scheduled an appointment with one of these two new oncologists. They got me in the next day. I would like to take credit for wisely becoming assertive at this point, but it was Genevieve who lit a fire under me.

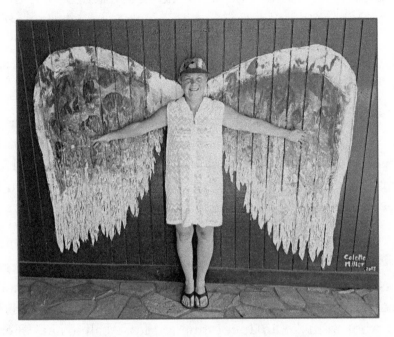

It helps to have an angel on your side
when the stakes are high.

That wasn't the last time that Genevieve was my best advocate. We met with this new oncologist the morning that I was to begin chemo. He told us that my insurance company had approved the use of two of the three chemo meds, but denied the third. That's when my sweet, loving, gentle Genevieve showed a side of her that you would never have known that she possessed.

Have you ever walked by a car in a parking lot with a dog inside? The dog has to defend his territory from lurking menaces, such as you walking by. Even a little three-pound

240

Chihuahua attacks the glass again and again, teeth bared, leaping at that glass one more time so he can break through and tear off your face. As you circle behind that car and slide over to your car door, this pup that is no bigger than a pastry snack looks more like ninety pounds of muscular pit bull. The glass starts looking a little more vulnerable. As the saying goes, it's not the size of the dog in the fight; it's the size of the fight in the dog. And YOU know he can't break the glass, but you keep eyeing all the car windows, sizing up the openings.

All this to describe Genevieve in the doctor's office. Her eyes were popping out of her head, her volume ratcheted up a few notches, and her skin flushed. She used the force of her "Kung Fu" voice (she's a brown belt) to inform the doctor that this was not acceptable. Although she made it clear that she was angry with the insurance company, not the doctor, he leaned back ever so slightly, and occasionally snuck a glance at the door. He looked as if he was wondering whether the car windows were rolled up far enough.

I suggested to him that we start all three meds, and sort out the insurance later. He immediately agreed to the plan, still with one eye on Genevieve. That's my little lotus blossom in action!

Further down the road, my track record with being my own advocate took another well-deserved hit. This new oncologist, whom I loved, also left the state. (What am I doing to chase the good ones clear across the country?) The clinic assigned a new oncologist to work with me. At least this time I checked his credentials, though not closely enough. I found out that he was a specialist in six different types of cancer. Now, we all know that if you specialize in one or two things, you can be a specialist. There is another name for "specializing" in a half-dozen cancers, however. It's called being a generalist.

I liked this new doctor, but he was clearly not a specialist. How was he going to know what options would be available to me when new treatments are coming out so fast that even genuine specialists are having a hard time keeping up? I should never even have gone to that first appointment with a doctor so unqualified for my needs.

It turns out that when my cancer started growing again, he didn't know of any options other than the same ones that had been around for decades: chemo and radiation. Surgery was not an option.

However, this time I was prepared. I told him about a clinical trial for a new cancer drug for people who progress off the medication I was taking. He hadn't offered this to me, because he didn't know it existed.

This time, being my own advocate saved my life. I got in the clinical trial. Now, twenty-five months later, the cancer has shrunk substantially, and my health remains stable. I am connected with a true lung cancer specialist for this clinical trial, and I'm not letting go.

These are all stories that show you how my passivity almost cost me my life, and how taking an active role in both my treatment and the choice of my treatment team saved my life. Many others have shared similar stories with me. Though not all resulted in life-or-death changes, each one shows the advantage of being your own advocate.

Sue, a friend who had Stage IV lymphoma, needed a hip replacement after cancer spread to her hip. She brought a friend with her to meet with the surgeon. However, the surgeon wouldn't look Sue in the eye. He stared at the floor, and occasionally glanced at Sue's friend.

This doctor had to leave the room for a minute. When he came back, Sue was lying on the floor.

"Are you alright?!" he asked.

"Of course," she said. "But this was the only way I could get you to make eye contact." Then she fired him, and found a doctor that suited her collaborative style better.

Is it any surprise that someone with that kind of attitude, who is willing to do whatever is called for to get the kind of treatment she needs, is still alive and cancer free, twelve years later?

It doesn't always go this well, however. My friend Jack had an excellent oncologist, who was part of an excellent team of oncologists. However, when his cancer started growing, he couldn't get his doctor to retest his genetic mutation, to see if there were any targeted therapy or immunotherapy options available to him. Instead, she gave him chemo. He wasn't comfortable getting a second opinion, for fear that he would get kicked out of the clinical trial that had already given him another year of life. This was his lifeline, and he feared letting go. By the time his doctor retested his genetic mutation, it was too late. Although he qualified for another clinical trial, he was already too weak to get on an airplane. He was gone within weeks.

The lesson here is that doctors may be brilliant, but that doesn't mean that their judgment is flawless, or that they would make the same choices that you would. You have to be your own advocate.

Charlotte, Genevieve's twin, was diagnosed with breast cancer. She took the mammogram to get a second opinion from a radiologist that she knew, one who was willing to go into great detail to explain the test results to her. Charlotte wanted to make sure that when she met with her oncologist to make a treatment plan she had a full understanding of the options.

Next, Charlotte interviewed an oncologist. "How would you treat this specific breast cancer?" she asked.

"With this type, I always do the same protocol. I do A-B-C-D-E."

"Always?"

"Yes, always."

Charlotte fired her, and found an oncologist that was more willing to work with her, as part of a team making collaborative decisions.

Another friend, Lysa, lives in a community that doesn't have any lung cancer specialists, and traveling to a more specialized clinic on a routine basis was not an option for her. She solved the problem by spending an hour or two every day on the Internet, doing her own research. She sends articles to her oncologist about promising treatments that may be a fit for her. Her oncologist, who is willing to collaborate, follows up on the research, and then discusses it with her at her next appointment.

Lysa also advocates for others, doing things such as research and going to appointments with them. Upon Lysa's suggestion, one of her friends asked her oncologist to have her cancer tested for genetic mutations, which is essential to take advantage of the treatments that have been coming out for the past several years. The oncologist was incensed that a mere patient thought she knew more about lung cancer than he did, and he refused. This person fired her oncologist. She found someone more open to collaboration, and who was also open to the newest, most effective treatments.

Jessie's doctor was willing to test her for only two genetic mutations, although there are at least three that have associated targeted-therapy treatments. When Jessie asked about a test that she had learned about for over 150 genetic mutations, her doctor said, "Absolutely not. You can't afford it, and it wouldn't change how I treat you anyway."

Jessie contacted the lab directly, and found out that they had a sliding fee scale, which meant that she could afford the test. She learned that she had a rare mutation, and took the results to a lung cancer specialist who is considered a guru in lung cancer mutations. This expert told her that one case with her mutation had been treated successfully for eight months in Spain, but pursuing it wasn't worth wasting her time.

Would it be worth your time to find a treatment that might extend your life? That's not a hard one for most of us to answer. The last time I talked to her, Jessie was trying to find someone to translate for her, so she could call the clinic in

Spain and find out what kind of treatment had been used successfully for her mutation.

All of these examples point to the same things, which are also this chapter's...

CHALLENGE EXERCISES:

1. Check the credentials of both your doctor and your clinic.

2. Make sure you have a lung cancer specialist. *A specialist in six different cancers is not a specialist.*

3. Get molecular testing. It's the only way to get treatment targeted for you.

4. If the cancer starts growing again, get molecular testing again. The results will not be the same.

5. Do your own research, either by piggybacking on what other survivors have learned, or looking at the data yourself.

6. Get a second opinion.

7. Make waves if you need to. It's worth risking hurting your doctor's feelings if it means that it may save your life.

8. Treat your doctor like he or she is your consultant, not your parent. Seeking your doctor's approval is not as important as getting the results you need.

9. Even if all of this is not your style, it's important to make yourself uncomfortable and do it anyway. Your life may depend on it.

RESEARCH

The best way to predict your future is to create it.

~ Abraham Lincoln

In the earlier years, I didn't spend any time at all looking at research on the Internet. Of course, there wasn't much new going on in lung cancer in 2006, so it didn't matter as much. I wasn't expecting an Internet search to make a lot of difference the second time I was diagnosed, but I couldn't have been more wrong. If I hadn't spent just enough time to get to know my buddy Craig online, I never would have found out about a clinical trial was about to close, a trial that saved my life. That got my attention: I am now much more diligent about research.

Where do you even *start* looking for the kind of information that you need? Here are a few suggestions:

See the table on "National Resources for Lung Cancer" at the end of this book. You will find almost anything that you are looking for, though it will take some time perusing to see what fits for you. Some have forums where you can ask questions about your specific circumstances, such as, "Has anyone been on Medication X? What can you tell me about it?" The cancer community is very generous about sharing information.

You can also link to @LCSM (Lung Cancer Social Media) on Twitter. This will tap you into links to research, trending ideas, and whatever else you may want to find.

It will also help if you find bloggers in a situation similar to yours who find it important to do their own amateur research, and to let others know about it. It may save you from reinventing the wheel.

Of course, *you* may be the person who wants to do the most thorough research accessible to the layperson. It is a valuable gift to the cancer community to gather this information and share it with others. This can be a blessing or a source of increasing stress, or perhaps both, so it is a good idea to pay attention to what impact doing this research has on you.

I hope you will keep in mind that the goal is to stay alive *and* to enjoy the life that you have. This will impact how much time you want to spend on the Internet.

CHALLENGE EXERCISES:

1. Find the table "National Resources for Lung Cancer" at the end of this book.

2. Find three of the resources that look interesting, and browse their websites.

3. Specifically, try out a few of the Clinical Trial Locators. Some are far more sophisticated than others.

4. If you are on Twitter, follow @LCSM.

PART IV:

SPIRITUALITY, GROWTH,

AND ACCEPTANCE

SPIRITUALITY

The Way is not in the sky; the Way is in the heart.

~ Buddha

I've touched on this elsewhere, but religion and spirituality are too important to ignore. Whether this is a topic on your own mind or not, it is very likely that many other people will press the issue.

For clarity, I am using spirituality to refer to one's *individual* belief system, while organized religions each have their own *shared* belief system about a higher being, with expectations and/or rules about behavior.

There are few things in life more personal than our spiritual or religious beliefs, or more threatening than someone else's beliefs if they are different from our own.

To add to this challenge, many religions consider it the responsibility of the faithful to get others to believe as they do. If the faithful fail at their mission, the souls of those that were to be converted are lost for all eternity. From this point of view, the only compassionate thing to do is to convince the other person to believe as you do, whether that person likes hearing about it or not.

If you are the other person and do not accept this point

251

of view, it is extremely uncomfortable to have someone ask about your beliefs and refuse to accept what you do not wish to discuss. How can you feel respected when you are told that you have missed the boat, and that you should think the way that the believer does?

This unsolicited help can actually make dealing with cancer more of a challenge. I have spent many hours thinking about how I can tactfully reply to people that have pressed me to accept their religious beliefs as my own. I take the time and energy to do this when I am able, because no matter how much I would prefer that they stop, I still believe that their intention is heartfelt. This tactful approach takes a lot of energy, and I do not always have the reserves.

Differing religious beliefs make for a great deal of friction. As an example, I received an email from someone who, in so many words, asked, "Now that you're closer to death, are you ready to accept Jesus into your heart?" I was stunned by the insensitivity of the question. Despite this, I still believed that this person's heart was in the right place.

I responded by thanking her for caring about me and sharing her very personal testimonial. I told her that my religious beliefs were different from hers, and that, while I chose not to share them with her, I requested that she respect my beliefs, just as I respected hers.

On another occasion, I sent out an email to family and friends in which I thanked them for their support "from the bottom of my soul." One person used this as a launching pad for a discussion of my soul, complete with Bible quotes. I chose not to respond. My energy comes and goes, and I don't always have enough left over to respond to what someone else deems important.

Still, even if I believe that the delivery is a bit awkward, I do my best to keep in mind that the intention of people who make these offers is honorable.

In the end, I don't think it matters which religion you believe in. Every form of spirituality that I have been exposed to, whether it is part of a formal religion or not, has features that I appreciate and respect. The less they are about rules, the more they seem to come from the heart, and the more I appreciate them.

I don't think I'll go to hell if I don't believe a certain way. I don't think I'll go to heaven, or have a better life the next time around, if I believe a certain way either. For me, there is something more important that is common to all religions: They're all about love.

I've had plenty of opportunity to think about this. Many people have prayed for me. I have had to ask myself: Do I care if they're praying for me in a church where their beliefs don't match my own? Yes, I do care. I am thrilled that they are praying for me. Do I mind if they're praying to the aliens? Not at all. Thank you for praying to the aliens for me. Am I OK with people sending positive thoughts my way instead of prayers? Please do. I love it.

I was deeply moved when my devout Catholic aunt told me that she had not only had a Catholic mass said for me, but that she had also gone down the street and made the same request at the Lutheran church. I'm pretty sure it was the first time she had been to any religious institution outside of the Catholic Church unless a wedding was involved. That meant a lot to me, because it came from her heart.

A family member asked me if I minded if she said a prayer for me in her particular church. While I appreciated being asked, I told her that if she was saying a prayer for me, I was going to take in the message. She was sending love my way, and I was grateful for that.

Prayers and positive thoughts may even change things in ways that we don't understand. I can accept this as possible too. Therefore, I appreciate prayers and positive thoughts even when I don't know that people are sending them my way. People have different beliefs about the afterlife, about the existence of heaven, hell, purgatory, or reincarnation. To me, it's not that complicated. It's all about love. The connection is very powerful and runs deep. What some may call God, I call sharing love with each other.

Just feeling this love will give me more strength and energy to continue in my battle. The more directly I know about it, the stronger the impact will be on my heart and on my health. The same goes when I share my love with others, and we both benefit.

My stepfather, Vince, has had an enormous influence on my growth and development since childhood, and he remains an influence on me even after his passing. All of us become immortal by influencing each other, hopefully in positive ways. We don't have to wait until we're dead for that to happen.

To me, when people send love to each other with their thoughts, words, or actions, it is spiritual. In the end, love is all there is.

CHALLENGE EXERCISES:

1. Think of one example of a time when someone pressed their religious beliefs upon you and wouldn't take "no" for an answer.

2. Write down how you might respond to that person in a kind yet assertive way. Although your words may be different, here is an example: "Thank you for encouraging me to accept your beliefs. While I know that this is very important to you and that your intentions are good, I have my own beliefs. I hope that in the future you will respect that I have made my own decision. I know that I can always come to you if I change my mind."

3. Role-play your response with a friend or loved one.

ACCEPTANCE

For after all, the best thing one can do
when it is raining, is to let it rain.

~ Henry Wadsworth Longfellow

Acceptance in any form is hard to come by, yet deeply rewarding as each new layer settles in. Some of these forms are unique to our current circumstances as survivors. Since there isn't a one-size-fits-all way to come to acceptance, the best I can do is to share my own experience of inching in that direction.

Let's start right out with the big one. I am accepting that I may die from cancer in the near future.

Before I could accept this possibility, I had to face it head on. I did the usual mental wrestling: If I accept that I may die, am I giving in? If not, will that make me the tough survivor who refused to accept what the doctors were telling him, and lived because I *didn't* accept it? Will I live longer because I am fighting death?

You have probably heard about some tough old buzzard who was "too mean to die" and who lived much longer than anyone could explain for any reason other than refusing to accept death. Maybe it's true, and if so my hat is off to these people. I have to say that it's not my style, however.

We all have to find a way to survive that works for who we are, and I believe that the approach that works best will be different for different people. I am convinced that there are many ways to do this.

I decided that the refusing-to-accept-death or too-mean-to-die approach is not a fit for me. I believe that if I'm going to survive, it will be for a different reason.

It will be because I love my life, and I want to keep living.

There is nothing contradictory about accepting the possibility of death and also loving life. There is also nothing contradictory about accepting the possibility of death and staying alive. In fact, I would argue the opposite. By accepting that I may die, I can let go of many of the fears that could otherwise dominate my outlook. How does hanging onto those fears leave any room for me to live or to enjoy life? How does that leave any room for me to grow?

In the words of Einstein: "You cannot simultaneously prepare for war and plan for peace."

This may sound like a one-time decision. It most definitely is not. It comes and goes. Anytime something new comes up with my health, the fear comes with it. However, the more times I face the potential progression of the cancer, the easier it is to let the fear in, accept it, and then let it pass through me. The fear doesn't stay as long, and acceptance of death goes a little deeper the more I practice it.

However, as you are no doubt well aware, we are not in

this alone. The people around us will have their own reactions, which can at times be a challenge in itself.

If you have been dealing with cancer for longer than a week, you have probably already seen that some people handle your news well, and others do not. Some people go out of their way to be a resource for you, and others will do their best to avoid you.

If you have spent any time reading cancer blogs, you will find many reactions, from both blog writers and those that comment on the blogs, about what are thought of as the shortcomings of people who don't have cancer. Those with cancer sometimes call the non-cancer people around them insensitive, selfish, or worse, and often with a lot more vinegar in their words. I understand this. Part of what we are going through is grieving the loss of our health, and potentially our lives. How then, we think, can people who do not have cancer that are close to us be seeming to be anything less than caring, at a time when we are going through the biggest challenge of our lives? The perceived lack of caring can be a stunning blow.

My own experiences have not been nearly as bad as those of many of the people whose stories I have read. The worst that I have experienced was to be avoided by some people, and to encounter others who offered no support other than the instruction to keep them informed – I'm dealing with cancer, and they are giving me a job to do for them?

My reference to grief is important, because one of the stages of grief is anger. It is much easier to get angry at someone who has hurt us than to cope with our own potential loss of life.

For most of us who have cancer, getting past this anger towards others isn't quick or easy. I can talk about this mostly in the rearview mirror because I have been fortunate enough to see it with the perspective of time. I'm here to tell you that you can come out on the other side with a rewarding sense of acceptance of these people, with all their flaws.

My sister-in-law Vicki got through this phase much quicker than I did. She was diagnosed with three different cancers in one year, and sent me an email on the one-year anniversary of her first cancer surgery. She was cancer-free and grateful for the changes she had experienced since she was first diagnosed. However, what really struck me was the following sentence: "I've learned who really has the strength to support me and those who do not, and I do not think any less of those who can't."

Wow! *That* was an impressive attitude for someone who had been diagnosed just a year before. Vicki had come to acceptance in a very short time, and it was clear from emails and conversations that it was real, and that her life was better because of it.

I hope that you too find a way to get through anger and come to acceptance. After all, it is the final stage of grief, and the one that brings the most satisfaction and fulfillment.

We have already talked about acceptance of the potential loss of your own life, and acceptance of how others act towards you. The last form of acceptance is the most rewarding, and that is another of the greatest of cancer's gifts.

The last form of acceptance is acceptance of yourself.

I think this is something that most of us struggle with and yet rarely talk about with others. But why shouldn't we? What could be more important? What could impact our daily lives more than being able to accept ourselves for who we really are?

None of us are going to be able to meet all the expectations that others have of us. Parents, siblings, partners, friends, coworkers, even strangers—we worry about a disapproving look, a perceived slight, a lack of recognition from any of these people. We are imperfect in just about every way, but we want people to notice only when we do something exceptionally well. Harder yet, we internalize what others think about us. As a result, we don't want to admit to being less than perfect, even to ourselves.

After a lifetime of being even more prone to feeling the need to be perfect than most people, I now find it a lot ~~easier~~ less hard to drop the perfection obsession and be who I am.

Multiple things have conspired to make this easier. When friends let me know that they want me to live, and go out of their way to let me know that they care about me, more of it sinks in. It's easier to feel loved, which makes it easier to love myself. When my appearance changes in ways that I don't like, and yet people still accept me as I am, that sinks in too.

Having potentially limited time also helps to put things in perspective. The brand of your shirt seems pretty irrelevant when you feel sick and your hair is falling out. Forgetting to pick up milk on the way home from work doesn't seem like a mistake worth beating yourself up over. You can let go of the need to please a family member that you have never been able to please, because your life is your own now. Losing a checkbook may cause some stress, but it doesn't need to cause self-flagellation.

The irony of possibly having limited time to live is that, now that you know it, you have more time to resolve your unfinished business. For me, that included letting go of who I thought I was supposed to become: the perfect father, someone who is comfortable spending a lot of time around people, a person with many passionate interests. I have had to accept who I am now, in this present moment, because there is no time left to become someone else.

It's not only accepting who you are, however. It's being kind to yourself, and doing things for yourself like buying new clothes even if you don't think you'll be around long enough to wear them out, and test-driving a new Tesla, and going to see the rose gardens in the spring, and leaving work early if you're too fatigued to get much else done for the day. It's accepting who you are. It's loving yourself.

For me, part of it has been accepting that the love of my life is with me every step of the way that she can be with me, but that there are also some steps that are mine and mine alone. She can't climb into the MRI tunnel with me, or experience the nausea from chemo, or face the possible end of my life as if it were her own. I have embraced those steps as something to be treasured, no matter what they are, *because* they are mine and mine alone.

The same is also true for you:

This is your very own experience. Treasure it.

CHALLENGE EXERCISES:

1. The next time the fear of dying hits you and you can't push it away, let it in completely. Let your thoughts take you where they will, without blocking any paths. Sit with the feelings until they pass.

2. Write down everything that you learned from this experience. Was it as hard as you thought? How did you feel when the feelings passed? How long did that feeling last? What did you learn about your fears? What else did you learn about yourself?

3. The next time someone angers or hurts you, even a little bit, by how they react to your cancer, ask yourself if the person tried to hurt you, or if it was something else, such as their ignorance or lack of social grace.

4. Reconsider whether what you are responding to is really your displaced anger at your own cancer.

5. List five situations in which you have been hard on yourself, and write down what you said to yourself.

6. Write a letter to the person that you love most in the world as if he/she were in that situation. This time, take each of those five situations and tell that person the most caring, nurturing thing that you would say if he/she were in that situation.

7. Replace that person's name with your own, and read the letter to yourself.

CONSIDERING CANCER AS A TOOL

There is no education like adversity.

~ Disraeli

I have found a lot of new coping skills, and strength I never knew I had. Buried in the details of this good stuff is realizing how much I have grown because of cancer.

The irony here is unsurpassed. While cancer attacks my body, I am growing. While some parts of me are being eaten up, other parts are thriving. While some parts wither, others are expanding.

Cancer has helped me become more open in many ways. Before, it was pretty easy for me to be dismissive if something wasn't in my frame of reference. As examples, I wouldn't have even considered that my thoughts and feelings could impact my health, and couldn't buy the idea that other people might be able to send healing thoughts/prayers to me. I would have dismissed the possibility that alkaline water could change my body's pH, and therefore help me beat cancer, out of hand. Although I still don't agree with that last one, I have given it careful thought.

To make sure that I'm seeing the whole picture, I have used my blog to ask friends and family why they think I am still alive eight years after first being diagnosed. About thirty of these important people offered their opinions. In broad categories, they included attitude, having a clear intention to stay alive, love (and also, specifically, love from and of Genevieve), support from others, God/spirituality, having a purpose on this planet, the right treatments, having balance, and luck. I wanted to listen carefully to each of their ideas, all of which I think are contributing factors, and some of which I might overlook if I wasn't paying close attention.

In my pre-cancer days, I never would have asked such an important question, because I wouldn't have wanted to hear conflicting opinions, and I would have felt too awkward if I disagreed with some of the responses. Now, I'm more willing to be accepting when someone has a point of view very different from my own, be it about world politics or miracle cures.

I'm doing a much better job of living in the present and staying engaged, rather than trying to "ride it out" so that I can get back to "real" living. I can even enjoy my time stuck in traffic, because instead of being impatient to get somewhere, I realize that I am somewhere already. I live in gratitude for just about everything around me. I am more accepting of different styles, perspectives, and choices, such as astrology, fundamentalist religious beliefs, things I would classify as "woo-woo," and people with unshakable prejudices. As a partial result, I have more respect for others.

I could also say that I'm more forgiving, but that wouldn't be true. What is true is that I find less in others that I feel might need to be forgiven, because I have become more accepting of people just the way they are. I am more courageous, particularly about sharing my life with others. I am more optimistic.

I have become more open to accepting love and support from others, and to giving it to others as well. Both parts of that equation have made it easier for me to love myself.

You get the idea. I'm telling you that cancer can be one of the greatest experiences of your life, even if none of us would volunteer for the job.

My friend Chaz told me that he had read somewhere that pessimists recognize a problem, and then see all the additional problems that will be created. An optimist sees the same problem, but sees the opportunities that the problem creates. Cancer has helped me become more of this kind of an optimist.

This is one of the things that I hope you will take from this book. Cancer can be a negative in your life, and there is no doubt that parts of it will be.

But cancer can also be seen as an opportunity, a tool for growth.

Cancer gives you an opportunity to connect more closely with the people that you care about, to heal old wounds. You can find your courage, and seek out the meaning in your life. You have the ability and the opportunity to grow in every way. All you need to do is be open and ready to take advantage of these new experiences when they come your way.

I hope you will find a way to make this experience your

own, to embrace it, and to live a full rich life.

This is the time.

This opportunity is one more gift from cancer.

CHALLENGE EXERCISES:

1. List five ways that your life has changed for the better because of cancer.

2. List five things that you can do that will make your life even better.

EPILOGUE:

BECOMING THE ANTI-ADRIAN

Everyone wants to live on top of the mountain,
but all the happiness and growth occurs
while you're climbing it.

~ Andy Rooney

Not long ago, Genevieve and I met with my oncologist to get my CT scan results. It was his last appointment of the day, and he looked as if he wished his day had already ended. This time, he said, the results were not good. The cancer was growing again. The targeted therapy had stopped working.

I was running out of treatment options. He scrunched his face and looked at the floor for much of the time while he went over the remaining options. It looked to me as if all hope was drained from his face.

"What about the clinical trial for Drug XYZ?" I asked.

"What clinical trial for Drug XYZ? I didn't know that was out yet!"

"Yes," I said. "It's in San Diego."

"But that's in San Diego!" he said. San Diego is a

269

thousand miles from Portland.

"That's right," I said.

As soon as I got home I called my friend Craig, who was already participating in this trial. He gave me the contact info that I needed.

The next morning I immediately got to work. I called *and* emailed the clinical trial coordinator, "Master of the Universe" (MOU) for my purposes, essentially telling her that I would do backflips and cartwheels, paint myself purple, and turn myself into a Wookie if it would get me into the clinical trial.

She emailed back to tell me that the clinical trial was closing to new participants the following Friday, which was seven days away. I would have to see a doctor within that time to get a foot in the door. However, she couldn't make an appointment for me until she received *all* my clinical records, biopsies, and scan results *for the last eight years*. And, by the way—wait for it—she would be... *on vacation* starting at 5:00 pm that day. I had the rest of the day to pull together all her requirements.

Next, I called my oncologist's office to grease the wheels of bureaucracy by using the two-pronged frontal assault, from both doctor and patient. However—wait for it—he was... *on vacation* starting that day.

About this time, my back was so tense that it felt like a coiled steel spring. If someone had snuck up behind me and said, "Boo," I probably would have jumped right over my desk. I might have even left a trail behind me.

I spent the day scrambling to get two hospital systems and two clinics to pull all my clinical records together. I also had to beg the hospital film libraries, both of which told me that it would take them a week, to treat this with more urgency. Those records would need to be on discs, which I would hand-carry to San Diego.

In the end, the pieces tumbled into place. Both OHSU and the Oregon Clinic got past their internal glitches and computer failures and faxed their small mountains of records to MOU, and both hospital film libraries told me that they would have my scans burned on CDs by Monday. At 5:30 pm, MOU emailed to tell me that my appointment would be on Tuesday.

MOU started her vacation right after hitting the "Send" button. But that is not the end of the story.

In the course of eight weeks, I flew to San Diego seven times. There was the initial appointment, the lung biopsy to make sure I had the right genetic mutation to be eligible for this trial (a 50/50 proposition), multiple EKGs, an echocardiogram, an eye exam, blood and urine samples, questionnaires, and a few things I'm sure I've forgotten. There will be three more appointments in the next two months. After that I'll make the trip only once every six weeks. There are no CT results yet, but it feels like I'm breathing easier already.

Why do I tell you all this?

Because it is important to me to urge you to make the most of your opportunities.

I am doing everything within my power to give myself the best chance to live for as long as possible. A number of people with cancer have told me that they would do "anything" to make sure that they lived longer. Yet when the challenge is presented, they decide too much is being asked of them.

In the early part of this book, I wrote about Adrian, who had lung cancer and was still smoking, and how I wanted to be the "anti-Adrian." This is me, being the anti-Adrian.

I found a clinical trial that will likely extend my life (yet again!), and I have jumped through every possible hoop to make sure that this opportunity didn't pass me by.

There are no guarantees, but so far it's working.

The message is the same for you. There are no guarantees that anything you do will extend your life. It is almost a given, however, that your life can be better if you make the most of your opportunities.

Cancer *itself* is one of those opportunities. My life has become much richer because of this experience. Coming close to losing my life has a way of making me treasure it.

I hope you realize what a treasure your own life is.

That is cancer's final gift.

TO BE CONTINUED

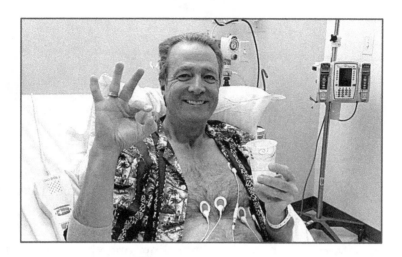

Victory smile: Starting the clinical trial.

ABOUT THE AUTHOR

Dann Wonser was first diagnosed with Stage III lung cancer in 2006. In these past twelve years, he has had two lung surgeries, two courses of chemotherapy, one alternative chemotherapy, radiation treatment, several minor procedures, and two targeted therapies, including one that was still in clinical trial. Now, he is a lung-cancer blogger at www.dannwonser.com, public speaker, and member of several national and local committees on lung cancer. He lobbies both state and federal congress for lung cancer issues. He has been a guest blogger for two national cancer organizations, appeared on radio and television, and serves as a featured lung cancer role model at www.lvng.com. He has taught self-advocacy to others through a workshop, and has been the subject of articles for national cancer magazines.

Throughout all of this, Dann has continued to work full-time.

Cancer has taught Dann lessons he never comprehended when he was earning his master's degree in counseling psychology, or in the twenty-five years that he worked in the mental health field. He has jettisoned the toxic relationships and other unhealthy influences in his life, and has more meaningful relationships with those he loves. His priorities have come into clear focus. He is happily married to an extraordinary woman, and his quality of life has never been better.

DANN'S TREATMENT TIMELINE: VERSION 1

There are two versions of this timeline. This version covers only diagnosis and treatment. See the following page for an alternative version that shows the full picture of what life has been like over these past eleven years.

July 2006: The first lucky break: Stage III lung cancer found by accident.

Aug - Dec 2006: Two rounds of chemo, then surgery, then two more rounds of chemo.

Jan 2007 - May 2011: No Evidence of Disease (NED) for four and a half years.

August 2011: Lung biopsy confirms Stage IV lung cancer.

Sept - Dec 2011: Four rounds of chemo. No shrinkage, but cancer remains stable.

Dec 2011 – June 2012: Treatment with a chemo maintenance drug. Cancer remains stable.

June 2012: Maintenance drug discontinued due to kidney damage.

June 2012 – May 2013: Despite no treatment of any kind,

cancer remains stable.

May 2013:	Cancer has progressed within lungs and spread to bones.
May 2013 – Sept 2014:	Treatment with targeted therapy reduces the cancer by 30 percent in my lungs in the first three months.
October 2013:	Two weeks of radiation therapy effectively reduces the pain to my hips.
September 2014:	Cancer found to be progressing in lungs again.
Oct 2014 – Present:	Accepted into clinical trial in San Diego. The cancer shrinks 60-70 percent in the first six weeks, and has remained stable through the time of this writing.
July 2006 – Present:	Living life in gratitude every day.

DANN'S TREATMENT TIMELINE: WHAT LIFE IS REALLY LIKE

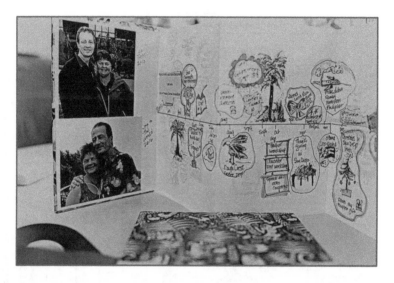

For most of our marriage, Genevieve has kept a timeline of our most memorable events of each year. Of course, she adds her own artistic touches. It has been a wonderful reminder of the richness of life.

NATIONAL RESOURCES FOR LUNG CANCER

Group Name	Website	Blog	Expert Blog	Inspiring Stories	Clinical Trial Finder	Info About Lung Cancer	
American Cancer Society	www.cancer.org			X		X	
American Lung Association	www.lung.org	X		X	X	X	
Bonnie J Addario Lung Cancer Foundation	www.lungcancerfoundation.org	X		X	X	X	
Cancer Grace	www.cancergrace.org		X			X	
Cancer Support Community	www.cancersupportcommunity.org	X				X	
CancerCare	www.cancercare.org	X				X	Additional information about these resources is on the following page.
Caring Ambassadors	www.lungcancercap.org						
Cure Today magazine	www.curetoday.com/tumor/lung						
Free to Breathe	www.freetobreathe.org				X	X	
HealthUnlocked	www.healthunlocked.com	X					
Imerman Angels	www.imermanangels.org						
Inspire	www.inspire.com	X					
International Association for the Study of Lung Cancer	www.iaslc.org					X	
Lung Cancer Alliance	www.lungcanceralliance.org				X	X	X
Lung Cancer Foundation of America	www.lcfamerica.org				X		X
Lung Cancer News Today	www.lungcancernewstoday.com						
Lung Cancer Social Media	www.lcsmchat.com	X		X		X	
Lung Force	www.lungforce.org	X		X		X	
Lungevity	www.lungevity.org	X	X	X	X	X	
Lvng With Lung Cancer	www.lvng.org			X			
National Cancer Institute	www.cancer.gov				X	X	

Group Name	Practical & Financial Resources	Helpline or 1:1 Peer Support	Facebook	Conferences	Articles / News	Other
American Cancer Society	X			X	X	
American Lung Association	X	X		X		
Bonnie J Addario Lung Cancer Foundation	X	X	X		X	
Cancer Grace						
Cancer Support Community						Also has a teen blog
CancerCare	X	X				Webcasts & podcasts. Also online support groups for caregivers, and for survivors
Caring Ambassadors						
Cure Today magazine					X	
Free to Breathe	X	X	X			
HealthUnlocked						
Imerman Angels		X				
Inspire						
International Association for the Study of Lung Cancer				X	X	Videos
Lung Cancer Alliance	X	X	X	X		Advocacy, Lobbying
Lung Cancer Foundation of America						Advocacy, Research
Lung Cancer News Today					X	
Lung Cancer Social Media						Topical Twitter Chats
Lung Force						
Lungevity	X	X	X	X	X	Research
Lvng With Lung Cancer	X		X			
National Cancer Institute					X	

CPSIA information can be obtained
at www.ICGtesting.com
Printed in the USA
LVHW030600220121
677170LV00003B/100

9 780999 635100